# Going the Distance

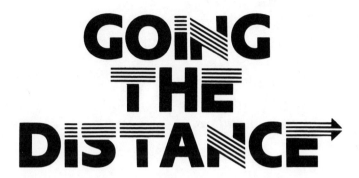

# GOING THE DISTANCE

## The Right Way to Exercise for People Over Forty

Ronald M. Lawrence, M.D., Ph.D.
Sandra Rosenzweig

JEREMY P. TARCHER, INC.
Los Angeles
Distributed by St. Martin's Press
New York

*To Eleanor, Michele,*
*Lesli, Stewart, and Allison:*
*For all their love*
*and support throughout the year.*

RON LAWRENCE

*To DBR:*
*Just for the halibut,*
*then and always.*

*to IMR:*
*One of two,*
*now and forever.*

SANDRA ROSENZWEIG

**Library of Congress Cataloging-in-Publication Data**

Lawrence, Ronald Melvin
  Going the distance.

  Bibliography.
  Includes index.
  1. Aerobic exercises. 2. Exercise for the aged. 3. Middle age—Health and hygiene. I. Rosenzweig, Sandra. II. Title.
RA781.15.L39 1987    613.7'1        86-23096
ISBN 0-87477-414-4

Jeremy P. Tarcher, Inc.
9110 Sunset Blvd.
Los Angeles, CA 90069

Design by Deborah Daly
Illustration by Valerie Deo

Manufactured in the United States of America
10 9 8 7 6 5 4 3 2 1

First Edition

# C O N T E N T S

CONTENTS

# ACKNOWLEDGMENTS

Every book is a group project —a collaboration of writers, editors, and agents with lots of help and patience from family and friends.

We especially thank our editors, Suzanne Lipsett and Janice Gallagher. Suzanne held our collective hand throughout the entire process, organizing, questioning, challenging, and clarifying both concept and style. Janice nursed us along, cajoling, encouraging, and directing us throughout, combining support and sensitive counsel with her special way of making every critique appear to be a compliment.

And then, there's our agent, Martha Casselman, with her savvy editorial and visual sense. Truly, she's the person without whom. . . .

# INTRODUCTION

# The Sweet Joys of Moving Around

Happy fortieth-plus birthday, and welcome to sports for fun and profit—profit in health terms, that is. *Going the Distance* takes the mystery, fear, and drudgery out of exercise for people past forty. We believe that if you choose the right kinds of exercise, you will become fitter, healthier, more energetic, and thinner. And the odds are you'll live longer, too. You'll feel better and you'll feel better about yourself. We offer you fourteen feel-good options—everything from walking in the sunshine to skiing in the house—and we promise you'll enjoy every minute.

## True Aerobics: Easy, Fun, and Health-Promoting

*Going the Distance* promotes back-to-basics aerobics—all those ways of moving that strengthen your heart and lungs, lower your blood pressure and harmful blood cholesterols, trim away fat, lift you out of depression, fill you with energy, add years to your life, and shape up your entire body.

We're talking true aerobics here—the only truly aerobic, anyone-can-do-them sports around: walking, running, cycling, swimming, rope skipping, cross-country skiing, rowing, canoeing, and kayaking. What's more, all of these sports, except canoeing and kayaking, are as fun and beneficial indoors as they are outdoors. You can exercise in the sun and fresh air, or you can exercise in the privacy and convenience of your own living room and still get all of the life-giving benefits of pure aerobic exercise.

You may be surprised to see cross-country skiing, rowing, canoeing, and kayaking here. They may sound like advanced, highly athletic, complicated sports, well beyond your abilities. They aren't. In fact, all of these sports are simple, easy, and quick to learn—our Five-Minute Lessons will get you going with no trouble at all. None of them takes any special athletic ability. All of them, including the skiing, are nice and safe. You cross-country ski by gliding and sliding along on flat ground wherever there is a little snow—none of that nerve-wracking whizzing down hills at breakneck speed associated with downhill or Alpine skiing. You row, canoe, or kayak on quiet, flat water—not on the white-water rapids you see in the movies. It's a shame these sports aren't better known. They are among the most aerobic, beautiful, exhilarating, slimming and trimming, and enjoyable sports around. And they're cheap if you rent the equipment from local sporting goods stores.

We want you to discover how easy it is to exercise, how much fun it is, and how wide your choices are. You don't have to be athletic to exercise. Neither do you have to enjoy punishing yourself. Exercise doesn't mean doing fifty boring push-ups or forcing yourself to run around your neighborhood. Aerobic exercise—our kind of aerobic exercise—is something you look forward to, and throughout the book, we'll give you hints about how to keep it fun for the rest of your life.

We're *not* talking about the so-called aerobics that's taken the country by storm in the last few years. As we'll explain in Chapter 2, no bouncing, kicking, bending, bounding exercise you do at a gym or health spa or in front of the television—be it a jazzy workout, "reducercizing," weight lifting with machines or free weights, or just plain thirty minutes of leg lifts, torso twists, and donkey kicks—none of these is noticeably aerobic, no matter what their teachers say. The good ones will tighten up your thighs and midriff, but they won't make you healthier.

Our sports will make your body firm, lean, and limber, and they'll help improve your health, mood, and vitality. The other exercises won't change your body chemistry (metabolism) to work faster and burn extra calories for the next four to six hours after you've exercised. Our sports will. The other exercises won't earn you several hours of renewed energy to carry you through the rest of your daily activities. Ours will. Those other exercises won't add years to your life. The sports in this book certainly will.

And best of all, all of the sports in this book are easy. You can learn them in just a few minutes by taking our special Five-Minute Lessons. It may take you a few days or even a few weeks to hone your skills, but you're not going to be gasping for breath or aching all over and wishing you could just sit down with your feet up. That's the big surprise about truly aerobic exercise. It's not supposed to be hard. It shouldn't take too much out of you. If it does, it's not aerobic. That familiar coaches' saw of "no pain, no gain" is hopelessly old-fashioned and dangerous.

Even better, our sports are fun to do. You're not going to get bored and count the seconds until you're done. People we know love doing our aerobics. They look forward to the relaxation and pleasure of exercising as much as they look forward to the results. We don't subscribe to the head-against-the-brick-wall theory of exercise. You know the one: it feels so good when you're done.

We assume that you want physical fitness without spending your whole life exercising. Our sports kill three birds with one stone: (1) you'll discover just how good you can feel; (2) you'll strengthen your heart and lungs, speed up your metabolism, and conquer depression; and (3) you'll firm up flabby muscles and limber up tight, achy joints. Why waste your time sweating and groaning with a class or a video for anything less?

You may wonder about a few omissions. "What?" you may ask. "No golf? No tennis? No bowling?" No. And no softball, volleyball, racquetball, or arm wrestling, either. It's not that we're turning our collective back on hard drives straight down the fairway or slashing forehands. It's just that this is a book about becoming healthier. Only aerobic exercise makes you healthier. Tennis, golf, bowling, and the rest are great fun and enormously satisfying, but they don't make you healthier because they aren't aerobic.

In order for an exercise to be aerobic, it must conform to some precise specifications.

1. It must make you huff and puff but only moderately. Too easy isn't aerobic. Neither is too hard.
2. It must be nonstop—no rest periods allowed except when you're just beginning. This is one of the most important requirements for aerobic exercise.
3. It must make you sweat.
4. It must use your large muscles (such as those in your thighs or shoulders).
5. It must use those large muscles to pull you across some distance. Jumping in place or within a small area counts for very little.
6. It must make those large muscles contract steadily, repetitively, and rhythmically throughout the exercise period.
7. It must last for a minimum of thirty minutes.
8. It must be done at least three days a week.

Let's see how some sample sports measure up.

*Golf* rarely makes you huff and puff and sweat. If you walk, you do use large muscles to pull you across a distance, but if you ride in a golf cart, forget it. Golf is definitely not nonstop; it is one of sports' original stop-and-start games, offering plenty of opportunity for rest. Yes, it does last more than thirty minutes. Whether it's played three or more times a week is up to you, but considering how poorly it rates otherwise, what's the difference?

*Tennis* usually makes you huff and puff and sweat and uses your large leg muscles to pull you across a distance, but even when played intensely, it's much too stop-and-start to contract and relax your muscles rhythmically or bring any aerobic benefits. Tennis buffs often ask us why they're not in good shape even when they play three times a week or more. Given the game's poor aerobic rating, how could they be?

*Dance exercise* makes you huff and puff and sweat and uses your large muscles in rhythmic and repetitive ways. But you don't cover ground, and you don't move aerobically for at least thirty minutes nonstop. (Even if the class or videotape lasts an hour, the actual aerobics—the getting up and jumping around part—usually lasts about twenty minutes. That's why the authors of the popular body-shaping and dancing programs tell you to walk or run a couple of miles after you finish their workouts.) Whether you dance exercise at least three times a week depends on how conscientious you are. (Note: Heartbeat, the focus and obsession of dance exercise instructors, is only one aerobic factor out of eight.)

How do the fourteen sports in *Going the Distance* rate aerobically? Admirably. Every one meets or exceeds all eight requirements. Even better, you're unlikely to get hurt using our programs. With the exception of running, the sports in this book are the ones with the lowest injury records. All in all, we consider them as close to perfect as any man-made activity can be.

Does this mean you should never play tennis again? Of course not. How could we deprive anyone of the joy of putting away an archrival with a perfect little drop shot just over the net? It simply means you need something else, something aerobic, in order to feel healthy and fit. *Going the Distance* is a health book. We want you to get into shape and stay there. Then you'll be playing some hot games of tennis with your pals when you're eighty.

# How to Use This Book

No matter how anxious you are to get on with the real point of this book—which is to exercise—read Part One first. It explains what aerobics is and why it is such a powerful tool for getting into shape and becoming healthier at the same time. And it tells you all you need to know about environmental considerations and, when necessary, medical considerations, to ensure that your exercising is safe and health-promoting. Here, you'll learn how to dress in hot or cold weather, how to warm up and cool down, how to stretch and how not to, and how to eat well for sports. You'll also learn what you need to know about exercise, sports, and the particular medical conditions often associated with the second half of life. With Part One under your belt, you can start any exercise program in our book safely and begin to feel results right away.

Parts Two and Three give you short but thorough courses in the fourteen sports we have carefully selected as particularly well suited to both beginners and advanced sportspeople age forty and up. Part Two, indoor exercise, shows you how to cycle, row, walk, run, jump rope, cross-country ski—yes, even ski—without ever leaving home. Part Three presents outdoor sports—walking, running, swimming, cycling, cross-country skiing, rowing, canoeing, and kayaking. You'll be able to follow these descriptions in the field. They'll walk you through everything from how to find a good pair of shoes to how to paddle a canoe to how to treat the few injuries you may encounter.

With our clear, uncomplicated, easy instructions, you can start at the beginning level, then progress through intermediate and masters levels at your own pace. We've designed programs to help you pace yourself week by week and get into shape and improve your health with no strain or pain. These gentle schedules are undemanding, medically sound, and completely safe for anyone over forty. Nothing could be simpler. And if you reach the advanced masters level, we suggest options to make exercising even more interesting—everything from bird-watching walks to luxury bicycle tours of France.

There's even something for the competitive souls among us. Most of the outdoor sports described in Part Three have national and international age-graded masters athletic programs. You swim, speedwalk, cycle, ski, or row in local, regional, and—if you get that far—national and international races against people within four years of your age (forty to forty-four, forty-five to forty-nine, and so on, up into the eighties). Each local chapter or team trains regularly, usually at public pools or the facilities of a nearby YMCA, YWCA, YMHA, or YWHA, and these classes are often the best places to learn the intricacies of your sport, whether or not you intend to compete. Write to the national governing bodies listed in the Resources section at the back of this book for the addresses of local chapters nearest you.

We even teach you how to perform each sport, starting with your very first steps, so you don't need any previous experience to begin. All you have to do is follow the special Five-Minute Lesson in each chapter. (The one exception is swimming. We do recommend official lessons for swimming if you really can't swim a stroke—not even a dog paddle—or if you're afraid of the water. Once you've got the fundamentals, we take it from there with a Five-Minute Lesson on how to swim effortlessly and efficiently.) If you choose to take lessons from a friend or an accredited instructor, our Five-Minute Lessons will still help you perfect your style with the insights and pointers we've developed over years of teaching people how to get moving.

Use *Going the Distance* as your pocket guide to the whole world of commonsense exercise. Read straight through to get a sense of your options; then settle on one sport or another and work out a personal program. Above all, experiment. Too many people consider their exercise programs to be grim, inflexible commitments. We urge you to discover how much fun exercise is. Then you'll do it because you enjoy it, not because you *have* to. It will relax you and make you feel better. In all exercise, you will uncover something of the marvelous about yourself. We hope *Going the Distance* helps you learn the sweet joys of moving around.

# PART
# ONE
## What You Should Know

In theory, you can start exercising without reading a single word about whether exercise works, how and why it works, and whether it's safe. Just lace on your walking shoes or climb on your bike and you're off.

However, most of us need reassurance. We want to be convinced. As one man said to us, "No way am I spending all that money on walking shoes just because someone told me it's good for me. You've got to prove to me that I'll feel better and you've got to swear to me that I won't hurt myself."

That's what the next four chapters are all about. You'll learn why doctors consider exercise to be the fountain of youth, the miracle cure, and the best route to a slim, trim figure.

After you've read Part One: What You Should Know, turn to Parts Two and Three to find your dream exercise—or two or three.

*Then* tie on your shoes and take off.

# Not Bad for Forty— or Fifty—or Sixty, Not Bad at All

**L**et's be frank. Chances are, you're not reading this book because you're just dying to exercise. You're reading this because you think you *should* read it. Perhaps you passed a mirror and thought, Do I know you? Or your doctor—or, worse, a friend—pointed out that you should be able to climb a flight of stairs without gasping for breath. Or you read yet another article about how people who exercise live longer, have lower blood pressure and fewer heart attacks, and are thinner, healthier, and more energetic than people who've gone soft and tired over the years.

First you want to be convinced: is it really true that exercise will make you feel and look better? And isn't there some easier way to achieve the same goals?

In answer to the first question, it is true that exercise will give you more energy and more zest for life, make you look thinner and healthier, and help you live longer. That's why people who exercise regularly are devoted to it. They love the great rewards they reap for such a small investment.

In answer to the second question, no: there is no other way

to get there from here. To understand why, let's look at what happens to your body as you grow older.

## "I Feel Better Than I Ever Have Before": The Paradox of Aging

Beginning in your early twenties, your body starts slowing down, especially if you are inactive. Your heart pumps about 8 percent less efficiently every decade. Fatty cholesterol deposits clog your arteries, so that by middle age, your coronary arteries are 29 percent more closed than when you were in your twenties. As a result, your blood pressure rises.

Your lung capacity decreases and your chest wall stiffens so you can't inhale as much oxygen. Therefore, you send less oxygen to your muscles, skin, and other organs. Without enough oxygen, your body tissues age more quickly. You look and feel older than you should.

Each decade, you lose 3 to 5 percent of your muscle tissue, so your arms and legs gradually lose their strength and speed. At the same time, you have a higher proportion of body fat to body muscle. In other words, even if you weigh the same now as you did at twenty, you're fatter.

By the age of seventy-five, your body can do less than half the work it could do at twenty. (Scientists measure this by calculating the amount of oxygen the body uses.) Your reaction time slows as your nerve cells age. Your bones lose their minerals, get soft, and break easily.

Cheer up: some things *improve* with age. Your wisdom, understanding, and experience become greater with every passing year, for example.

You may read bleak predictions of bodies slowing down, clogging up, and wonder, "How can this be? I feel better than I ever have." Many of you, in fact, may find you feel better and better the older you get. Maturity brings greater self-respect and self-acceptance.

You feel good about yourself when you're in control, and one of the best ways to take control is to improve your health and physical appearance. In fact, your own body is one of the few things you can completely control. So you make a pact with yourself to look the best you can. Forget about looking twenty again. Instead, you promise yourself: Within two months, I will be able to feel proud of myself and boast, "Not bad for fifty-five. Not bad at all!"

# Aerobic Exercise: The Fountain of Youth

Exercise and heredity sit on opposite sides of an invisible see-saw. Your heredity determines how and when you age. You'll live about as long as one or both of your parents. Your hair will gray when theirs did. You'll probably get arthritis or high blood pressure if one of them did.

Exercise is the only thing that changes this process. With exercise, you won't feel your arthritis nearly as much as your mother did. You won't have to take as many drugs to lower your blood pressure. You'll be hiking through the Sierra foothills at seventy, an age when your father could barely walk up the stairs. Exercise is still the only fountain of youth known to humankind.

But we're not talking just any old exercise here. We're talking *aerobic exercise.* What can a good aerobic exercise program do for you? Let's take it point by point (see Chapter 2 for details).

\ *Aerobic exercise can give you the stamina and health of someone almost half your age.* Middle-aged runners, for example, have a cardiovascular fitness level only 14 percent lower than that of trackmen in their early twenties—a 4 percent decline per decade instead of the usual 8 percent.

*Aerobic exercise makes your skin glow and your complexion vibrant because it improves the circulation to your skin.* Hence, you look younger.

*Aerobic exercise seems to protect against heart attacks.* For example, longshoremen in a study of 6,300 San Francisco dockworkers had half as many deaths from sudden heart attacks as those with more sedentary jobs. The conclusion was that hard physical labor each day protects people from heart attacks. This seems likely, because the number of heart attacks among longshoremen started going up when mechanization and containerization hit the shipping industry and lightened the workload. Another study, this one of 36,500 men at Harvard University between 1916 and 1950, showed that men who burned at least 2,000 calories a week in strenuous aerobic exercise had one-third fewer heart attacks than those who played golf, bowled, or did not exercise at all.

*Aerobic exercise lowers blood pressure,* thereby lowering the risk of heart attack, stroke, and even the memory loss and mental changes that often accompany fatty-cholesterol buildup in the arteries of the brain. Aerobic exercise also thins the blood plasma, the liquid part of the blood. (Thicker-than-normal plasma has been found in people with rheumatoid arthritis, tuberculosis, and even some cancers.)

*Aerobic exercise opens the tiniest arteries and helps build new ones* to protect you against heart attack.

*Aerobic exercise lowers the level of bad cholesterols in your bloodstream.* There are good, neutral, and bad types of cholesterol. Exercise increases the amount of good cholesterol, which scrubs out your arteries and removes the bad artery-clogging cholesterol. As a result, exercise not only lowers the amount of bad cholesterol in your bloodstream but often eliminates some of the cholesterol plaques already blocking your arteries.

*Aerobic exercise helps dissolve blood clots that might cause heart attacks and strokes.* The exercise provokes your body to stimulate the production of plasminogen, which dissolves fibrin, the stringy protein that forms blood clots.

*Aerobic exercise improves your digestion and regulates your bowels* by speeding up the muscular movements of your intestinal tract.

*Aerobic exercise helps you lose fat and keep it off forever—something no diet can do,* because it regulates your appetite so you eat only when you're hungry. It also helps unhealthily thin people put fat on their bones by *stimulating* their appetite.

*Aerobic exercise helps smokers quit smoking.* It's not a surefire cure—nothing is—but exercise sometimes reduces the craving for tobacco. Smoking makes the heart pound faster, narrows the blood vessels and raises the blood pressure, reduces the amount of blood sent to the heart, and lowers the amount of oxygen in the bloodstream. Those smokers who breathe deeply only when they take a nice long drag on a cigarette will find that their huffing and puffing during a brisk walk gives them the extra oxygen they crave. Exercise also prevents the new nonsmoker from gaining weight. Smoking makes the body burn 10 percent more calories than it would otherwise. Quitters who don't do something extra to burn calories—exercise!—will start to fill out in all the wrong places.

*Aerobic exercise hardens your bones to prevent or reverse osteoporosis* (thin, brittle bones). Although osteoporosis is a serious problem for older, postmenopausal women, it affects younger women and men too.

*Aerobic exercise is a reliable cure for depression, on-the-job stress, nervousness, confusion, and the overall jitters*—better than any drug on the market. As you walk or cycle or whatever you choose, you bring more oxygen to your brain, and that makes you more alert. Your chosen exercise also breaks down excess adrenaline and other stress-produced chemicals stored in your brain and heart. As you exercise, your brain produces endorphins, sometimes called the brain's opium, which relax you, relieve nervous tension, and make it easier for you to sleep soundly at night.

*Aerobic exercise makes you more mentally alert.* It gives you more energy because you've taken in so much more oxygen. It also improves your concentration and boosts some sorts of memory and reasoning processes.

*Aerobic exercise attacks women's monthly blahs. It minimizes premenstrual syndrome and may cure menstrual cramps, probably by a combination of mechanisms.* If you're in shape, your muscles are strong, and strong muscles don't cramp up as easily. When you exercise, you warm up your muscles, and warm muscles usually uncramp. The endorphins you release during exercise may relieve premenstrual tension and mask menstrual pain. And exercise may inhibit prostaglandins, a group of chemicals produced in the body which, among other things, stimulate cramping in the uterus and other muscles.

*Aerobic exercise is the most valuable ally women have during menopause.* It may reduce hot flashes, and it certainly encourages sleep. Insomnia, which dogs many women during menopause, accounts for a lot of the notorious menopausal crankiness. The endorphins produced during exercise also soothe menopausal irritability. Exercise prevents weight gain and boosts self-image.

*Aerobic exercise may release a natural infection fighter, endogenous pyrogen, in the body, helping to prevent colds and other illnesses.*

*Aerobic exercise reduces most sorts of pain because it stimulates production of endorphins to mask discomfort, it produces chemicals to inhibit prostaglandins, and it warms up the muscles.* It improves just about any condition you can think of: varicose veins, rheumatoid arthritis (exercise works better than any drug), cervical degenerative arthritis, lumbar-sacral arthritis, diabetes (exercise may reduce the amount of insulin needed), low back pain, night cramps, prostatic hypertrophy, asthma and other lung diseases, ulcerative colitis, stomach and duodenal ulcers, and some kinds of cancer.

*Aerobic exercise often interrupts even severe headaches in mid-torture.* It also prevents migraine, tension, and other types of headaches. The headaches you do get are fewer, farther between, and weaker when they hit. Note: migraines are the exception. Once in full swing, they become more painful with exercise.

Have we left anything out? Well, exercise can improve your sex life by giving you more energy and more stamina and by toning and limbering up your muscles and joints. It may also clear up adult acne. (In all honesty, however, it's also possible that exercise will make acne worse. Some acne reacts badly to sweat and sunshine.) Exercise also speeds recovery after surgery, and makes you feel proud of yourself.

On the other hand, beware of all the self-congratulatory magazine articles promising salvation through exercise. They profile superpeople who are lean and athletic, never overeat or overdrink, and never miss a workout. Because they are so physically fit, they are smart, organized, successful, competent, attractive, dynamic, youthful. They are go-getters, great leaders, and top salespeople.

This worship of the religion of physical fitness is just a phase, and it too will pass. Exercise serves only one purpose. It makes you feel good. If you put this book down now and never so much as walk across the living room, take this thought with you: you're not a jerk. You're just someone who's missing out on a good time and some good health.

# What *Is* the Right Way to Exercise?

Aerobic exercise changes our bodies from the inside out, making us fitter, more energetic, and healthier. Still, let's face it: in the short haul, we're more concerned about how we look than how we feel. We figure if we're going to put in that kind of effort, we want to come out looking firm and being able to touch our toes without groaning.

## What Aerobics Isn't

Theoretically, aerobic exercises don't sculpt our figures or limber up our joints. Theoretically, all they do is strengthen our hearts, lungs, and circulatory systems and trigger improvements in our body's chemistry. Firmness comes from strengthening exercises—a strong muscle is a tight, toned muscle—and flexibility comes from stretching exercises to loosen too-tight muscles and joints.

That's theory. In fact, no exercise does just one thing—

conditions only your heart and lungs, say, without strengthening some muscle or other. It's difficult to walk without using your legs or to swim without using your arms. If you use your legs or arms, you strengthen and/or limber them.

Our type of aerobic exercise gives you all-around physical fitness. You'll discover just how good you can feel, strengthen your cardiorespiratory system, firm up flabby muscles, and limber up tight, achy joints.

As we said briefly in the Introduction, we consider the so-called aerobic exercise classes to be a waste of time. You don't get a big enough return for all the effort you put out. It doesn't matter what they're called—exercise dancing, aerobic-jazz, calisthenics, shaper-uppers, workouts with or without weights, or weight training whether or not it claims to be aerobic—the best they can do is tone and limber up your muscles. They can't give you any of the other rewards of feeling physically fit. If you want to feel really good and become healthier, you've got to go out after your exercise class or video and walk, swim, or do something else genuinely aerobic anyway. Why not save time and combine all of your exercise?

We realize we're bucking a national trend and savaging a multimillion-dollar industry. Still, no matter what the exercise teachers and video makers say, "aerobic" exercise workouts are not as aerobic as walking, swimming, cycling, or any other of the fourteen indoor and outdoor sports in Parts Two and Three of this book. They get your heart racing, they get you huffing and puffing and sweating, but there's a lot more to aerobics than that.

Add to that the fact that most of these programs are about as much fun as a torture chamber. You sweat and strain, body aching and wracked with pain, and what do you get? Sometimes firm thighs. More often, a backache or bad knees or a groin pull. Some of the most popular exercises are dangerous. Double leg lifts are death on the lower back; neck rolls may damage the neck vertebrae; many types of sit-ups hurt the lower and middle back; locked-knee bend-at-the-waist toe touches attack the lower back, along with every joint between your back and your foot; and the list goes on.

Overall, the high-impact, bouncing, jumping, and kicking so-called aerobic dances are the worst. They've caused an epidemic of injuries to the toes, feet, ankles, knees, and hips and made a lot of sports medicine doctors rich. Many "aerobics" instructors and their students have moved into soft or low-impact "aerobics" in the hope that these will cause fewer injuries. They don't; they just cause different injuries. High-impact "aerobics" is famous for shin splints, stress fractures, and tendinitis. Low-impact "aerobics" causes back strain, shoulder pulls, knee and ankle damage, and sudden pulls and tears. Many of the movements are unnatural, always a surefire source of injury. In addition, the back strains come from tensing and stretching beyond normal flexibility. The shoulder pulls result from flailing and overextending the arms to try to get the heart pumping quickly. Knee and ankle damage occurs when the body weight stays on one leg at all times (the alternative to bouncing and jumping and high-impact injuries). Many legs can't take all that weight when the knee is bent.

None of this seems worth the trouble. High-impact "aerobics" is very strenuous but not terribly aerobic. Low-impact "aerobics" aren't even as aerobic as the high-impact stuff—the less impact, in this case, the less aerobic effect. Why bother?

# What Aerobics *Is*

Ask ten people on the street how to do aerobic exercise, and nine of them will tell you to get your heart pumping quickly and that's all there is to it. But "aerobic" doesn't mean "high heart rate." It means, according to the *Random House Dictionary of the English Language:* "pertaining to or caused by the presence of oxygen." When sports doctors talk about "aerobics," they're talking about the chemical changes that take place in your tissues when they're loaded with oxygen. It takes more than a fast heartbeat to do this.

An exercise is aerobic if it meets *all* of the eight criteria listed in the Introduction. To be aerobic, an exercise must be in the middle range of exertion—not too easy, not too hard. And that depends on your own physical condition, not on how many miles you run or how fast you swim a lap. If you're breathing quickly but easily, if you're covering ground, and if you're moving for thirty to sixty minutes without stopping—this leaves out tennis, ballroom dancing, and racquetball—you're working at your own ideal aerobic pace.

As you get into better shape, you'll just naturally move

faster because your beginning pace will come to feel too easy. That's why we've included intermediate and advanced techniques for each sport. Keep your exercise moderate. It's safer, healthier, and much more aerobic that way. Overdoing it is a waste of time—unless you like shin splints, aching muscles, and, perhaps, the risk of a heart attack.

# What Aerobics Does

It all goes back to that dictionary definition: "pertaining to or caused by the presence of oxygen."

Your body works best with a high oxygen intake. You can get that amount of oxygen only by breathing deeply while being active. You must move. When you become sedentary, your body learns to adjust to lower amounts of oxygen, but it adjusts by compromising a lot of body chemistry. Aerobic exercise resets your body back to its ideal level.

## TAKE A DEEP BREATH: IMPROVING YOUR LUNGS AND HEART

As you get back into shape, a chain reaction takes place. Let's start with the lungs. When you exercise aerobically, you breathe faster and deeper. As you get into better and better shape—and it takes only about six weeks of training before your heart and lungs show marked improvement—your lungs hold more and more air. You don't take as many breaths during exercise as you did before. The exercise gets easier, and you recover more quickly afterwards.

Your heart and lungs are a team, making up the cardio (heart)-respiratory (breathing) system. Your lungs send their oxygen-rich blood to your heart, which pushes oxygenated blood to every one of your muscles and organs. As you get into better shape, your heart gets stronger, the muscular walls of the heart's main pumping chamber enlarge, and your heart then pumps more blood with each beat. Thus it can beat fewer times. All in all, your heart doesn't have to work as hard. A well-conditioned heart may beat twenty times fewer per minute. That's 72,000 beats fewer each day; more than 26 million beats fewer each year. That adds years to its life . . . and yours.

## TAKING THE PRESSURE OFF:
## YOUR BLOOD VESSEL NETWORK

Your arteries widen and become more elastic in order to carry this new larger flow of blood, and you grow new tiny blood vessels called capillaries. In other words, you have more and larger blood vessels. (Your heart and blood vessels together are called your cardiovascular system. Vascular refers to blood vessels.) As a result, your blood pressure goes down and, again, your heart doesn't have to work as hard.

The effect on your blood pressure carries through in your daily life. A study at the Human Performance Laboratory in San Francisco compared two groups of students. One group was assigned to a fourteen-week aerobic exercise program; the other did no exercise. The blood pressure, muscle tension, and anxiety levels of both groups were measured before and after. The students who exercised recorded lower blood pressure, less muscle tension, and lower anxiety levels than the sedentary group.

Having successfully de-stressed one of the groups, the researchers tried to pile the strain back on. They gave each group a test full of unsolvable problems but they didn't tell them the problems were unsolvable. They told them that the test results would indicate how well the students would do in college. When the researchers told the sedentary group that they'd done poorly on the test, the students registered higher blood pressure, anxiety, and muscle tension, as you'd expect. The exercising group also showed more muscle tension and anxiety but didn't show any higher blood pressure. Aerobic exercise, apparently, had helped these students handle their stress better.

## MORE POWER TO YOU: YOUR MUSCLES

When you exercise regularly, your bone marrow produces more red blood cells, which carry the extra supply of oxygen. This extra oxygen travels to your muscles. Your muscle cells respond by producing more mitochondria, the chemical power plants inside each cell. The muscle cells can then extract much more oxygen from your blood. The muscles take this oxygen and combine it with fatty acids, proteins, or muscle sugars to manufacture carbon dioxide, water, and ATP (adenosine triphosphate), the fuel that runs your muscles.

Muscle sugar gives your muscles quick energy, but there's not much sugar in each muscle. When it's gone, your body searches for another fuel. A trained body recycles the sugars it burns and turns for fuel to the fatty acids stored in rolls of fat—belly, hips, thighs, wherever there's plenty to draw on. An untrained body can't switch to fat very easily. In that case, when your muscle sugars give out, your muscles give out, plain and simple. When you're in good shape, you don't cave in as easily. You also burn up fat as you move. And that means you get thinner.

## TRIMMING THE FAT:
## LOWERING YOUR CHOLESTEROL LEVELS

Aerobic exercise reduces the amounts of dangerous fats that float around in your bloodstream. Of the various blood fats, high levels of cholesterol and triglyceride are associated with heart disease. Lowering your blood cholesterol improves your odds against heart attack by 25 percent.

However, it's not that simple. There are good, neutral, and bad cholesterols, and nobody yet has completely explained the role triglycerides play in all of this.

Cholesterol is a fatlike substance we need to stay alive. Our bodies use cholesterol to make many essential chemicals and tissues, such as cell walls, vitamin D, hormones (including sex hormones and cortisone), the sheaths covering nerve fibers, and the bile acids that help us digest fat. Cholesterol also makes up most of the plaques, fatty deposits that clog up our arteries and cause heart disease. We all hear about how important a low-fat, low-cholesterol diet is. What we don't hear is that our livers make 75 to 80 percent of the cholesterol in our blood. Only 20 to 25 percent comes from food.

There are three kinds of cholesterol. *"Neutral" cholesterol,* or Very Low Density Lipoprotein (VLDL), is the lightest cholesterol. It serves mainly as the grocery bag. It carries fat from your food or your hips to your body cells. Your muscle cells burn this fat as fuel to keep your heart pumping and your legs moving.

*"Bad" cholesterol,* or Low Density Lipoprotein (LDL), is a little heavier and forms the large, clumpy, fatty particles that help form plaques. This sludge sometimes gets massive enough to choke off the blood supply to the heart or brain, resulting

in a heart attack or stroke. The more LDL you have, the greater your chances of suffering a stroke or heart attack.

*"Good" cholesterol,* or High Density Lipoprotein (HDL), is the smallest yet heaviest of the cholesterols. It is also the least fatty. HDLs act as biological Drano to carry LDLs away from the arteries. In other words, neutral cholesterol carries energy-giving fats *to* the cells; good cholesterol carries bad cholesterol *away* from the cells. The more HDL you have, the less chance you have of suffering a stroke or heart attack.

Liproproteins are compounds made of blood proteins, cholesterol, and triglyceride. *Triglycerides* are fats and oils, plain and simple, the very same you eat in salad dressing. Some of the triglycerides in your bloodstream come from your food; the rest come from your liver. If you have high levels of blood triglyceride *and* high levels of bad cholesterol, your chances for some blockage in your arteries are greatly increased. If you have high triglycerides and only moderately high or normal levels of LDL, your chances for a heart attack or stroke may or may not be increased; the evidence is uncertain.

If your LDL and/or triglyceride levels are high, your doctor will put you on a low-fat, low-cholesterol diet. Unless you have some genetic aberration in which your liver produces too much triglyceride, losing weight and eating less fat and oil will help to bring your triglyceride level back to normal, but that diet will be far more effective if you combine it with regular aerobic exercise.

To lower your blood LDL levels, eating less cholesterol and saturated (solid) fat and more polyunsaturated and monounsaturated (liquid) fat should make a big improvement.

Equally as important, you want to raise markedly your levels of good cholesterol (HDL), because the good cholesterol sweeps away the bad. Exercise, not diet, is the most effective way to achieve high HDL levels. The next most effective tactic is to be a woman, since women, for some evolutionary reason, have higher levels of HDL. However, this is something not all of us can manage. Third in order of effectiveness is to quit smoking, if you're one of those who haven't already stopped. Fourth is to lose weight, which exercise also helps you to do.

Evidence shows that diet alone isn't nearly as effective as diet and exercise to lower bad cholesterol in the bloodstream. The most interesting evidence comes not from human beings but from our closest primate cousins. A surprising number of monkeys and gorillas in American zoos have died of strokes and/or heart attacks. Autopsies showed fatty blockages in their arteries. This surprised the scientists because these primates had lived all their lives on low-fat, low-cholesterol, vegetarian-fruitarian diets—the ultimate Pritikin diet. If they ate so well, where did the fatty plaques come from? And why don't their relatives in the wild have the same extensive blockages? Obvious answer: the gorillas in captivity didn't exercise. The free-ranging ones did.

Women on birth control pills take note: Researchers at Stanford Medical Center have found that regular aerobic exercise offsets some of the negative effects of oral contraceptives. The Pill is known to raise triglycerides and lower HDLs.

## PROTECTION AGAINST BLOOD CLOTS

Just a single session of aerobic exercise makes it much harder for your blood to form dangerous clots in your blood vessels, clots that could lead to a heart attack or stroke. When you exercise, you manufacture something called plasminogen activators. Plasminogen activators stimulate the production of plasminogen. Plasminogen dissolves fibrin, a stringy blood protein that collects into clots. The effect of one exercise session doesn't last for long, but regular aerobic exercise four or five times a week keeps the protection going all the time.

## THE MIRACLE "DIET"

Aerobic exercise helps you lose weight and keep it off. If you keep your weight within a healthy range, you have less risk of heart attack, high blood pressure, and adult-onset diabetes.

Exercise helps you lose weight in five ways:

1. Exercise itself burns up calories.
2. Exercise causes you to burn up extra calories for a few hours after you're done exercising by speeding up the chemical reactions in your cells.
3. Exercise burns fat for fuel, so it taps into your overly cushioned thighs, midriff, hips . . . or wherever you're built, let's say, too substantially.
4. Exercise builds muscle. Muscle tissue is working tissue, so it burns calories. Fat isn't working tissue, so it doesn't burn calories.
5. Exercise resets your appetite. It makes you feel hungry *only* when your stomach is empty.

## DEM BONES: STRENGTHENING YOUR BONES

Aerobic exercise, along with any other exercise that moves your body against gravity, makes your bones thicker, heavier, and stronger. That means that aerobic exercise protects you against osteoporosis, the epidemic of thin bones that makes more elderly people bedridden than any other disease. When you lift your leg up to take a walking step, for example, your muscle pulls against the bone. The bone responds by building a callus, just as your foot, when you walk barefooted, builds a callus to protect your tender skin. In this case, your bone absorbs calcium to toughen itself. The same thing happens when you lift a tennis racket to serve the ball. In fact, the playing arms of tennis players have thicker bones, as well as muscles, than their nonplaying arms. You have to strengthen every bone separately, however. Walking won't thicken the bones in your arms. And swimming, alone among all the aerobic exercises, doesn't do much for osteoporosis because it doesn't set your body working against gravity.

## MOOD CONTROL

Aerobic exercise is a marvelous tranquilizer, more effective in reducing muscle tension than the prescription tranquilizer meprobamate, more commonly known as Miltown. It reduces anxiety and helps you sleep better. The extra oxygen in your brain deserves some of the credit, but there's more to it than that. Aerobic exercise also breaks down excess adrenaline and the other stress chemicals you produce throughout the day.

What's more, your brain, spinal cord, and some of your glands (pituitary, adrenal, pancreas) show high concentrations of endorphins when you exercise vigorously. (You don't have to exercise purely aerobically to crank out the endorphins. Weight lifting, Nautilus, aerobic dancing—any sweaty activity —seems to start them flowing.) Endorphins, sometimes called the brain's morphine, are actually many times more powerful in relieving pain than morphine. They also help you learn and remember; counteract depression; relax you and relieve nervous tension; and make you feel good about yourself. They make it easier for you to sleep soundly at night, which helps you deal with your problems during the day. The more you exercise, the more endorphins you manufacture and the better you feel. Endorphins, in fact, may be the source of the all-too-rare "runner's high," that sense of extraordinary well-being that some runners brag about.

Just fifteen minutes of aerobic exercise also doubles the body's level of norepinephine, a hormone your brain produces whenever it's time for you to feel joyous.

## BUILT-IN VACCINATION

Regular aerobic exercise may also release endogenous pyrogen, a chemical that wards off colds and infections. Endogenous pyrogen, produced by your white blood cells whenever you start to get a cold or flu, tells your brain to raise your body temperature to fever pitch to fight off the infection. Strenuous exercise may raise your temperature to 102 degrees Fahrenheit, which may knock out flu bugs. This may explain why people who exercise claim they get sick less than they did when they were sedentary. Nevertheless, it is not a cure-all. No one should try to cure a 101-degree with a five-mile run.

## BUILT-IN PAINKILLER

Whether it's due to endorphins or to the fact that exercise widens blood vessels, aerobic exercise is a wonderful painkiller. Among other things, it relieves cluster headaches. (For those of you lucky enough not to get them, these are sudden, excruciatingly throbbing headaches that often attack the whole of one side of the face and last for hours or days, coming and going several times a day—with only short periods of relief in between—for weeks on end. They afflict men almost exclusively.) Cluster headache sufferers know instinctively that exercise will make them feel better. Many people in mid-attack will have the urge to pace around the house or go for a walk. Migraine sufferers, in contrast, don't dare move a muscle. Even twitching a finger sends waves of pain through their bodies. Aerobic exercise does help prevent migraines as well as cluster and tension headaches.

## AND WHAT ABOUT SEX?

Making love is strenuous but not aerobic. It does take some effort, however, and the better shape you're in—the stronger your muscles are and the more stamina your heart has—the better you perform. Exercise also increases your sex drive. A mere twenty minutes of exercise by someone in good condition causes the body to release sharply higher levels of testosterone. Testosterone is the male sex hormone but women have it too, just as men have some of the female hormone estrogen. Testosterone gives all people—male and female—their sex drive. Take it from there.

# The Aerobic Miracle

You'll see results immediately. You'll feel energized after your first walk. You'll feel looser and stronger after your first week. You'll look slimmer after the first month.

After only six weeks, your cardiovascular system (heart, lungs, and circulation) will show measurable improvements. A little before the three-month mark, you'll start losing noticeable amounts of body fat. After three months, your endurance and the amount of oxygen you can absorb will increase markedly. However, it takes about nine months for the bad cholesterols (LDLs) to drop and the good cholesterols (HDLs) to rise. But once these changes start, they continue as long as you continue exercising.

## WEEKLY TOTALS AND REWARDS

*Forty-five minutes* of stretching each week (fifteen minutes a day, three times a week) may be enough to prevent osteoporosis, but not to reverse it.

*One and a half hours* of aerobics each week (thirty minutes each day, three times a week) may:

- change compulsive Type-A personalities (with a high risk of heart disease) into easy-going Type-Bs
- fight depression and anxiety, lower blood pressure and cholesterol
- change body chemistry to make it easier to lose weight (you actually lose about three ounces per week without dieting)
- reduce the insulin needs of some diabetics.

*Two hours* of aerobics (thirty minutes each day, four times a week):

- *strengthens and rebuilds* bone in people with osteoporosis
- raises good cholesterol (HDL) levels
- reduces risk of a first heart attack by 20 to 25 percent compared with sedentary people.

*Two and a half hours* of aerobics (thirty minutes each day, five times a week) works off half a pound of fat per week *without a bit of dieting.*

*Three and a half hours* of aerobics (sixty minutes each day, three times a week, plus an easy half hour on a fourth day, for example, *or* forty-five minutes a day four days a week plus an easy half hour on a fifth day):

- lowers risk of a first heart attack by 35 percent, but
- doubles or trebles the risk of sports injuries, such as shin splints, tendinitis, and sprains.

Three and a half hours of aerobics is a lot. Anything more than that is overkill.

# C  H  A  P  T  E  R  3

# Safe and Healthy: Exercising Intelligently

When you were seven, you didn't stop to wonder whether running was safe or whether you were cycling properly. You just raced out the door and did whatever entered your head.

Wisdom and experience have taught you to think before you thwim. You want to be certain that it's safe for you to exercise before you try any of the sports in Parts Two or Three, and you want to know the most efficient, effective ways to do the most in the least amount of time. That's what the next three chapters are all about.

## Should I See My Doctor . . . ?

Most books and magazine articles contain the following disclaimer: Anyone over the age of thirty-five should see a physician before embarking on *any* exercise program. This is in line with the cautious approach of the American College of Sports Medicine. They figure that anyone under thirty-five who has no known coronary heart disease risk factors or previous history of cardiovascular disease may begin an exercise program without a special medical checkup. Anyone over thirty-five should have a checkup first. In either case, they advise starting any exercise program cautiously and gradually.

In fact, many sports doctors admit to one another that they themselves wouldn't get so much as a routine checkup before they started exercising. They, of course, have a pretty good idea of their own health, but they also know that if they start out slowly and gently, without strain, they're unlikely to hurt themselves. It is rare for exercise to hurt anyone, but authors and publishers make their disclaimers to prevent possible lawsuits in our litigation-happy society.

So the answer to the question whether you should see your doctor, then, is . . . maybe. If you are the average, healthy person, you are not likely to have a heart attack from doing any of the sports recommended in this book any more than you are likely to have a heart attack from going to a movie. But if you or your doctor has any cause to believe there's a problem, ask for advice before you start exercising. If you haven't seen your doctor recently, or if you're a man over forty or a woman over fifty, and if you haven't exercised recently, yes, you should see your doctor.

## How Much Should I Exercise?

When people ask this question, what they really mean is, "How little exercise can I get away with?" We'll answer the first question in good faith, and, in the process, you'll get an answer to the second question.

We suggest you try to exercise for at least a half hour at a time. According to the exercise physiologists, it takes eight minutes of aerobic exercise before the exercise even starts to benefit your heart, lungs, circulatory system, and muscles. If you exercise for only fifteen minutes, say, you're not getting much payoff for your effort.

Try to keep your exercise at a slightly sweaty, slightly huff-and-puff level. Any exercise, no matter how laid-back, will eventually give you some benefit, but if you want to feel all those wonderful aerobic changes, you have to get your body working. If you are puffing slightly but can still hold a conversation with a friend or sing a song, you're perfect.

If you want to know whether you're working at a nice, moderate aerobic level, ask yourself: am I smiling? If you are, you can't possibly be working too hard. (Makes you wonder even more about those grimacing runners you see every day.)

Try to exercise at least three days a week; four is better. Anything less than three days a week won't stimulate your body to improve.

Unless you are doing something very unstrenuous, exercise every other day instead of two or three days in a row. This gives your body a chance to recover and build you up stronger than you were the day before. (When you exercise, you actually tear some tiny muscle fibers. In the next twenty-four to forty-eight hours, your body repairs these fibers, protecting you by building them thicker than they were originally. That's one reason muscles get bigger as they get stronger.)

No matter how much you love your exercise, do *not* do it more than five days a week. Your body needs that time to recover and rebuild. If you overtrain, you tear down muscle without building it up again.

The quick answer, then, to how much you should exercise: at least a half hour at a time, no less than three and never more than five days a week, at a pace that makes you huff and puff but still lets you smile.

# Preparing Your Body for Exercise

## WARMING UP

Don't you love it when someone creeps up behind you and shouts "Gotcha" in your ear? Well, that's what you're doing to your heart and muscles when you start exercising without warming up first. Warming up is so important, we have included instructions for warming up in every sports chapter (Parts Two and Three).

Before you exercise at your usual brisk pace, you've got to get your circulation going, raise the temperature in your muscles and tendons and loosen them up, release the synovial fluid that lubricates your joints, and gradually adjust your heart to the extra movement.

It takes a minute and a half or two minutes for your aerobic system to click on. In the meantime, nature has provided you with a backup system—a kind of fuel that burns without oxygen. You have just enough to carry you until your aerobic system kicks in. There's only one rub: this nonaerobic fuel loads your muscles up with a waste product called lactic acid. If you work your muscles too hard during these first two minutes and produce too much lactic acid, your muscles will cramp and ache. (This is the "burn" that Jane Fonda tells you to go for.)

Unless you enjoy pain (and the possibility of a heart attack), it makes sense to start slowly every time you exercise. Get all the systems operating at full power before you turn on the steam. Otherwise, you'll feel like our friend who brought home a new exercise bike, hopped on and pedaled furiously for about fifty seconds. That was it. He couldn't go on. When he wasn't looking, someone had shoved a cactus down his throat and wrapped his legs in blocks of concrete. He returned the bike to the store. Nothing was worth that kind of pain.

When you're in good shape and warm up gradually, you don't build up enough lactic acid to notice its effects. But if you start out at full tilt, as you do in a race, or if you do strenuous exercise where it's hard to start slowly, such as running or jumping rope, or if you're not in good condition yet, you may get winded. Your throat will feel dry, your muscles will become heavy, and you'll wonder how anyone could say this is fun. You've accumulated lactic acid and it's going to take anywhere from two to fifteen minutes for your body to flush it away. Then, all of a sudden, you breathe easier, your throat is moist again, your muscles loosen up, and you feel energized. Now your aerobic system is working unencumbered. You've gotten your second wind. (Yes, there really is such a thing. It's a light, gentle relief and a sense of airiness.)

We urge you to warm up slowly. It's much safer. But as you get into better shape, you may want to sprint or race, and it's reassuring to know there is a second wind waiting for you. If you're in excellent condition, you may get your second wind in a couple of minutes; if you're in poor condition, it may take ten or fifteen minutes.

Warm up by moving around at an easy pace for about five minutes. In most cases, this means doing whatever you're going to do for exercise—walking, rowing on a machine, swimming laps—but slowly, gently. Once you're breathing a little faster and you feel looser and slightly sweaty, pick up the speed and get on with your exercise.

## STRETCHING OUT

For years, popular wisdom has proclaimed that we should stretch after we warm up our circulation and muscles or we'd pull muscles or tear tendons. Also, consensus declared that being flexible prevented back and neck problems.

Our experience says otherwise. We're convinced that stretching before most exercise loosens and relaxes your muscles just when you need them to be strong and stable. This is a controversial position, but recent studies show that warm-up stretchers hurt themselves more frequently than people who save their stretches for after their exercise. Also, in his practice, Ron has found that the most flexible patients have the worst back pain. It appears that stiff and strong people are better adapted to exercise than loose, weak ones. (Remember, muscles tighten up as they become stronger.)

However—and this is an important exception—if you're doing something that requires you to reach or bend far beyond your usual range of motion, you should do warm-up stretches to lengthen and loosen your muscles *before* you start your activity. (That's why dancers spend so much time stretching before they do any real dancing.)

Even if your activity doesn't require the limberness of dancing or throwing the javelin, you may be one of the minority of people who benefit from stretching right after they've warmed up and before their real workout. If you need stretching, you'll either feel tight and stiff while you exercise or you'll feel stiff for at least four hours after your workout. In this case, do a set of our No-Stress Super Stretches (see following section) after your five-minute warm-up and before you plunge into your actual constitutional. If you still feel tight during your exercise, stop after ten or twenty minutes and stretch again.

Most of us, then, should save our stretches until we're done exercising. If you're part of this majority, do them during your cool-down, or do them to relax you before bedtime, or do them throughout the day. But do them.

Make stretching a daily habit. In fact, make it almost an hourly habit. If you don't stretch, you'll get tighter as you get older. Stretch every day, and you can be as limber as a child. Whenever you feel tight or tense, stretch—even if you're sitting in your chair at the office. Raise your hands above your head and reach for the ceiling. Slowly twist your torso. Gently turn your head from side to side in slow motion. Roll your ankles clockwise several times, then counterclockwise. Roll your shoulders back a few times, then forward. You'll be amazed at the difference these small movements make.

Whenever you stretch, stretch correctly. A good stretch is slow and effortless. Reach just until you feel the *tension release*, then hold for a count of twenty to sixty seconds. If the stretch starts feeling too easy, reach a little farther, then hold for another twenty seconds or so. Don't stretch beyond what's comfortable. You should feel like a cat stretching after a nap, not like a contortionist in a sideshow.

*Don't bounce, swing, or do fast exercises.* This applies to any exercise, be it stretching or toning or anything else. Reach until you feel like you're stretching, then stop and hold. Bouncing tightens and shortens muscles instead of loosening and lengthening them. Bouncing also tears your muscle fibers. Swinging and speed give you momentum. If you swing your arms in fast circles, for example, the force of the movement pulls your back farther than you would otherwise reach. This isn't a natural stretch, and you're likely to pull something. In addition, swinging, like bouncing, tightens your muscles instead of stretching them. Any time you see teachers in a class or on a television program or videotape thrusting and twisting like frenzied disco dancers, ignore them. Reach with your stretch and hold it while they bounce. It's much safer and you get more stretch.

## No-Stress Super Stretches

These six stretches work miracles. You can do them individually, whenever you feel like it, or all together in a five-minute sequence.

These are not the usual stretching exercises. They are safer than just about every popular stretch you've been taught —there's no pulling, yanking, compressing vertebrae, or over-bending. (Among the dangerous stretches you see every day are: neck circles; shoulder stands, yoga plows, or bicycle pumping; waist circles; toe touches; hurdler or flamingo thigh stretches; splits; Chinese or Japanese splits; yoga triangle or yoga dog pose. As an aside, we also warn you against doing such toning exercises as straight-legged sit-ups or sit-ups with your legs anchored; double leg lifts; and jackknives—they're very dangerous for all but the strongest backs.)

The No-Stress Super Stretches stretch you more effectively than most popular stretches. In the bend-over-and-touch-your-toes sort of hamstring stretch, for example, you start out stretching the backs of your legs—somewhat—but as you try to bend farther and farther, your back muscles take over and you wind up with a limber back rather than looser hamstrings.

These stretches, in contrast, isolate the area you want to stretch. You can't cheat—a hamstring stretch stretches your hamstrings and that's it.

These stretches are designed so that anyone can do them and get great results. You don't have to be flexible in order to start them, the way you do for yoga and several other types of flexibility exercises, and you'll never outgrow them. These same stretches will limber you up and relax you throughout your life.

## NECK TILTS

- Let your mouth fall open a bit and gently bend your head forward so that your chin moves near your chest (see Figure 3.1). Don't let it actually touch the chest, though. Hold. That should stretch the muscles in the back of your neck.
- Then, keeping your head and eyes forward, angle your head a little to one side as if you were cocking your ear in order to hear better. Hold. That will stretch the side of your neck.
- Move to the other side—not too far—and hold.
- Finally, move your head halfway between the first and second positions to stretch the place where your back and side muscles meet.

Always keep your jaw relaxed, mouth slightly open, and your eyes focused in front of you. After a few weeks, when

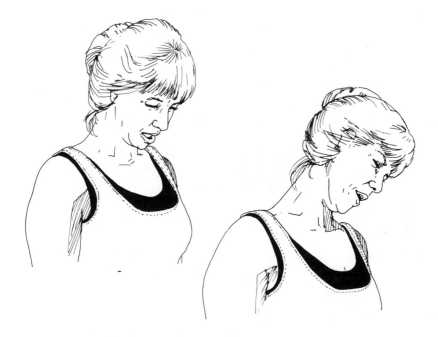

FIGURE 3.1    NECK TILTS.

you're used to stretching your neck, you can use your opposite hand to help pull your head—gently, gently—just a little farther. You don't ever want it to go very far.

In standard neck rolls, your head travels too far in every direction—ear tries to touch shoulder, head hangs so far back that you can't swallow, chin falls forward onto chest—and you compress your vertebrae and, once in a great while, rupture a disk. These stretches are much safer.

## BACK STRETCH

- Lie on your back on the floor—carpeted or not, but stay away from cushiony couches or beds.
- Bend your knees.
- Reach forward with both hands and grasp one leg *behind* the knee. (If you hold the top of your knee, you may put too much stress on it.)
- Bring the knee toward your head as you bend your neck and back to meet it.
- Try to touch your nose or forehead to your knee (see Figure 3.2). Hold.
- Repeat on other side.

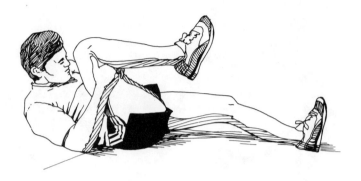

FIGURE 3.2   BACK STRETCH.


When this gets too easy, lie on your back with two pillows under your head. Grasp both legs behind the knees. Keep your jaw relaxed and your mouth slightly open. Pull your knees up as you bend your neck and back to touch the outsides of your forehead to the insides of your knees (see Figure 3.3). Hold.

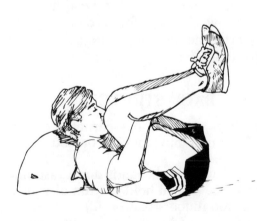

FIGURE 3.3   BACK STRETCH (ADVANCED).

## SIT-DOWNS

These are not stretches—they're toners, more bluntly called strengtheners—but as long as you're already on the floor, you might as well do them. We don't believe in body-shaping exercises, but we do believe in sit-downs. Even people in the best aerobic condition need sit-downs because they tighten and strengthen the abdominal muscles far more effectively than the standard sit-up and they don't injure the back. Strong stomach muscles are extremely important—not only to make you look good but also to prevent backaches.

- Start from a sitting position, knees very bent, arms across your chest, chin tucked down onto your collarbone.
- Suck in your stomach muscles and slowly, slowly lie down, curling backwards on your spine one vertebra at a time.
- As you roll back toward the floor, bend your knees more and more, bringing your feet closer and closer to your body (see Figure 3.4). Keep those abdominal muscles tucked in at all times. They will want to bulge out. Don't let them.

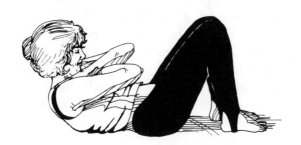

FIGURE 3.4  SIT-DOWNS.

- When you get to a midpoint, start sitting back up. That midpoint may feel as if it's halfway up your spine, or it may feel as if it's just before your shoulders touch the floor, or it may feel as if your neck is about a hand's spread from the floor. You'll recognize it because your stomach muscles will start to quiver if you try to stop and hold your position there. Move very slowly. The slower you go, the harder it is.

Standard sit-ups don't work and are dangerous. Don't do straight-legged sit-ups. Don't do sit-ups with your legs hooked under something. Don't do fast sit-ups. Don't do sit-ups with your hands locked behind your head. When your legs are straight or hooked under something, you use your hip flexors (also called iliopsoas), not your abdominals, to pull you up. Because the hip flexors run from the front of your thighs back through your pelvis to the small of your back, straight-legged and anchored sit-ups pull on the small of your back—not good unless you are dying for back trouble. What's more, you're not trimming your abdomen; you're tightening your hip flexors. Fast sit-ups use momentum, not abdominal muscles, to get you up and down. When your hands are behind your head, you use the momentum from your arms, as well as speed, to sit up. Again, no abdominals.

While we're at it, we'll warn you against double leg lifts. They are supposed to tighten your abdominal muscles, but they do that only if you keep your lower back pressed into the floor, which is next to impossible. If your abdominals are so weak you have to tone them up, they're too weak to keep your back pressed into the floor. When you do leg lifts incorrectly, and most people do them incorrectly, they arch and strain your back. In addition, don't do jackknifes, a seated version of leg lifts. Same reasons as above. Stick with the sit-downs.

Don't do waist circles. They are supposed to stretch your waist while trimming your spare tire. In fact, they damage your lower spine the way neck circles harm your neck vertebrae, and they stretch and weaken the side and front abdominal muscles, the very ones you're trying to tighten up.

## GROIN STRETCH

- Sit on the floor and bring the soles of your feet together in front of you. At first, just getting the soles of your feet to meet should be enough stretch.
- When that gets too easy, lean back so your weight is on your hands behind you, and lift your buttocks so that your knees come closer to the floor (see Figure 3.5).
- When that gets too easy, grab your feet, keeping your elbows out to the side, and slowly and gently bend forward (see Figure 3.6). Hold each stretch.

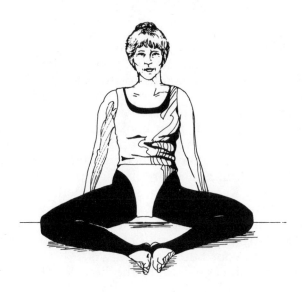

FIGURE 3.5 GROIN STRETCH.

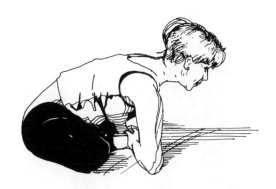

FIGURE 3.6 GROIN STRETCH (ADVANCED).

Don't do splits, so-called Chinese or Japanese splits (legs wide apart while you bend forward), yoga triangle or dog posture, or any other stretches based on standing with your legs as far apart as you can stretch them. Because they overpull the groin muscles, they actually tighten the muscles on the insides of your thighs—tighten them enough to tear.

## HAMSTRING STRETCH

- Stand up.
- Tuck in your stomach and relax your jaw.
- Bend your knees a lot, so that you can slowly bend over and touch your hands to the floor (see Figure 3.7). If you're practically squatting and still can't touch your hands to the floor easily, raise the floor by putting a couple of thick books under your palms. Throughout this exercise, keep your mouth slightly open, your chin almost touching your chest, your belly sucked in, and your rib cage pressed against your thighs. Keep one leg, say your left, bent, and slowly straighten the other. You probably won't get it very straight, but that doesn't matter. The point is to feel a stretch from well below your knee all the way up into your butt, and you will.
- Keep your rib cage close to the bent leg. Hold.
- Then bend the right leg and slowly straighten the left. Hold.
- To stand up, keep your abdominal muscles in, and uncurl, vertebra by vertebra, from your butt to your shoulders. Don't straighten your legs until your trunk is upright.

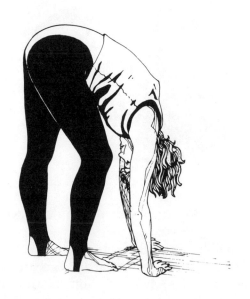

FIGURE 3.7  HAMSTRING STRETCH.

Don't do old-fashioned toe touches. They may pull the muscles in your lower back.

## FRONT THIGH (QUADRICEPS) STRETCH

Remember Mercury, the winged messenger symbol? While doing this exercise, you're going to look a little like him, except you'll probably be wearing more clothes.

- Pick a surface that comes up to about the middle of your thigh—a table or desk, the back of a sofa or chair, or the hood of a low-slung car.
- Carefully lift one bent leg, say the left, up onto the table. It doesn't matter how you get your leg up there as long as you don't fall and you don't arch your back.
- Now, swivel around so that your back is to the table. This leaves you standing on your right leg, with your back to the table, your left knee resting on the table, and your left foot sticking up in the air.
- Suck in your gut, and lean forward so you feel like a cartoon of someone running. Don't arch your back when you lean forward.
- To stretch, tighten your buttocks muscles, bend your

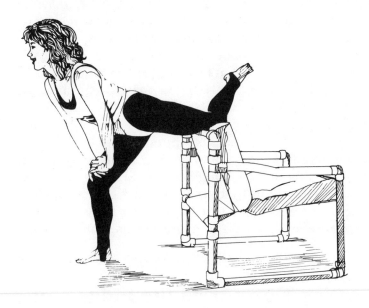

FIGURE 3.8 FRONT THIGH STRETCH.

right leg a bit, and, with your hands, push down on
your right thigh (see Figure 3.8). Hold.
• Repeat with other leg.

Many runners believe devoutly in the hurdler's stretch
and the standing thigh stretch to stretch their quads. (In the
hurdler's stretch, you sit on the floor with one leg bent behind
you, flat on the floor, and the other straight out in front. In the
standing thigh stretch, you grab one ankle and pull your leg up
behind you so you look like a flamingo.) Forget them. They
overbend and squash your knee and may tear the ligaments
holding your knee together.

## CAUTION

There are thousands of stretching exercises out there and most
of them feel delicious. However, a few are dangerous.

**Don't do any exercise with locked elbows, knees, or other
joints.** Locking strains your ligaments, the fibrous bands that
hold your joints together. It's okay to straighten your arms and
legs. Just don't lock them. To tell the difference, stand as
straight as you can. Tighten your knees, tuck in your buttocks.
Everything below the waist is now locked. Now, relax your
ankles, knees, and buttocks. That's what straight feels like.

**Don't do any exercise that overbends knees, puts weight
on knees while they're bent, or squeezes them tightly while
they're bent.** That means don't sit on your knees geisha fashion
and don't do deep knee bends. If you do, you may strain your
ligaments and tear your cartilage.

**Don't do yoga plows and other kinds of shoulder stands
(including old-fashioned bicycle pumping).** They are even
more dangerous than neck rolls because the full weight of your
body is stretching and pressing your spine along your neck.

**Don't do anything that arches back.** No back bends, no
gymnastic bridges, no dance or yoga poses. They squeeze the
disks of your spine enough to cause permanent and painful
damage.

## Cooling Down from the Inside Out

When you're done exercising, slow down gradually over five or
ten minutes to lower your heart rate. Do whatever you did to

warm up: pedal your bike at an easy pace, walk, do a lazy backstroke. Your heart needs this slacking-off period. While you exercise, your heart pumps huge quantities of blood to your arms and legs. Your muscles, as they move, push the blood back to your heart. When you stop moving, there's no way for the blood still trapped in your arms and legs to get back to your heart and brain. If you stop abruptly, all that blood pools in your muscles and you may faint or develop dangerous, abnormal heart rhythms. Five minutes of a slow jog, a slow paddle, or a slow pedal are all you need.

After you've tapered off the exercise, consider finishing your cool-down with the No-Stress Super Stretches. If your sport is one that feels like an effort, you'll probably need to stretch or you'll be sore afterwards. On the other hand, if you never get sore, you don't need any cool-down stretches. But they sure do feel good.

# Warning Signals

If you haven't exercised in years, or if you remember runner Jim Fixx's death with fear and trembling, you no doubt are worried that you might hurt yourself. It's natural to be concerned, but there's almost no chance you can get hurt doing the sensible types of sports presented in Parts Two and Three.

Sudden cardiac death during or after exercise has been much in the news but is actually extremely rare. Terence Kavanagh, medical director of the Toronto Rehabilitation Centre, did a statistical study of high-risk heart patients. These were all people who already had some sort of heart trouble. He reported that, as of 1985, there was only one fatal ventricular fibrillation (one sort of heart attack) for 214,777 hours of exercise, and only one nonfatal ventricular fibrillation for 367,000 hours of exercise. When he compared these statistics with the higher incidence of ventricular fibrillations among high-risk patients who didn't exercise, he concluded that it's much riskier to be sedentary than to exercise.

Still, as a smart exerciser, you should know the danger signals, so you will know if and when something is worth worrying about.

*See your doctor immediately (someone else should drive) if:*

1. You feel short of breath, clammy, or nauseated, and/ or have a squeezing or burning pain across your chest or deep under your breastbone or in the pit of your stomach or radiating into your upper back, jaw, arms, or hands. Exercising makes it worse. Don't delay. You may be having a heart attack.
2. You feel pain or tightness in the center of your chest or in your arm or throat during or after exercise. Stop exercising immediately. These symptoms indicate either poor circulation in the heart or a heart attack.
3. You feel light-headed, dizzy, confused, faint, out of control of your muscles, have the cold sweats, or turn blue. These symptoms indicate that your brain isn't getting enough blood. In the car on the way to the doctor, lie with your feet up or sit with your head down between your legs.
4. You get crushing chest pains at the beginning of exercise but they pass quickly, only to return a little while later. Your heart may not be getting enough blood. This could signal angina or a full-fledged heart attack.
5. You feel palpitations in your chest or throat, a fluttery pulse, a sudden drop in your pulse, or a flurry of rapid heartbeats. These symptoms may indicate abnormal heart rhythms.
6. You become extremely breathless for more than ten minutes after you stop exercising.
7. Your heart beats very, very rapidly for longer than ten minutes after you've stopped exercising.
8. You feel severe pain from any injury.

*See your doctor soon if:*

1. You have persistent pain in a bone, joint, or muscle due to a fall, blow, wrenching, tearing, or twisting.
2. You suffer joint pain that doesn't heal in two weeks.
3. You suffer an injury that doesn't heal within three weeks.
4. You experience any skin infection that shows pus, red streaks, swollen lymph nodes (often called glands), or fever.

*See your doctor if self-care doesn't help if:*

1. You are extremely tired twenty-four hours after exercising or if you develop insomnia (assuming you don't usually have trouble sleeping). You have probably overexercised. Try reducing the intensity or the length of your exercise.
2. You come up with a stabbing, searing, or aching pain during exercise in the top of your shoulder and neck or in your side or upper abdomen under your ribs. This is a stitch, caused by a muscle spasm in your diaphragm, and is not serious though it hurts like crazy. For self-treatment, see Chapter 11.

Now that you know how to handle your inner environment when you exercise, let's move on to how to deal with the environment outside your body—the heat, cold, sun, and rain.

# At Home with the Elements: Dressing to Beat the Heat and Cold

**S**o far, it may have seemed as if you're going to exercise in a sealed chamber, free from wind, chill, sweat, and wet. Many a walker or bicyclist, pouring sweat into the bright, eighty-degree August afternoon, has wished someone would invent such a chamber, but for the time being, we're stuck with the weather. When it's glorious, we're grateful for the chance to be out in it. When it's less than sensational, the best we can do is use it to our advantage when we can, and avoid it when we can't.

## Cooling It in Hot Weather

Obviously, hot weather makes us hot. Exercising also makes us hot, even in cold weather. Usually, we cool ourselves so efficiently that the extra heat doesn't matter. However, very humid or very hot weather interferes with our normal processes, and, if we're not careful, we turn into ovens and literally cook the protein in our tissues. As with a hard-boiled egg, once a heat injury has cooked part of our brain or heart, we can't uncook it. That's why heatstroke is so dangerous.

Individuals vary in how well they handle heat, but all people handle it less and less well as they get older. Somewhere around age sixty-five or seventy, the physiological responses to heat (and to cold) slow down. You don't realize you're hot, so you don't turn on the fan. Overweight people suffer in heat because that thick layer of fat acts as a built-in sweater to hold the heat in. People with heart disease, stroke, or diabetes also have trouble adjusting to heat. Several drugs interfere with the body's thermostat, slow down sweating, and interrupt the messages that signal overheating. Among these drugs are the phenothiazines (such as Compazine, Mellaril, Stelazine, Thorazine, Tindal, Repoise, chlorpromazine hydrochloride), and other anticholinergic drugs used to control vomiting and nausea, reduce motion sickness, increase heart rate, calm the emotions, and relax the muscles of the bronchial tubes, bladder, and bowel.

## PREVENTING HEAT INJURY

There are many symptoms of heat injury: excruciating muscle cramps; headache; nausea; fatigue; an odd sensation that you've got a lingering cold; inexplicable anxiety; heart palpitations; breathlessness; dim or blurry vision; dizziness; chills and goose bumps; feeling faint; numbness in hands or feet; rapid pulse; low blood pressure; gray, clammy, cold, wet skin.

If you notice the first signs of heat injury, STOP. Lie down in the shade. Put your feet up, about a foot higher than your torso. Apply cool wet cloths all over your body or douse yourself with cool water. Drink lots of cool water.

When you think about heating and cooling your body, imagine that your body is divided into two parts: the interior or core, made up of your heart, lungs, brain, and abdominal organs; and the shell, made up of your skin, muscles, arms, and legs.

Our bodies have two automatic, very efficient cooling mechanisms. When we get hot, the hot blood in the core of our bodies spreads to the skin to be cooled off. We sweat, and the sweat evaporating off our skin cools us off. Second, when the warm blood hits our skin, the blood vessels near the skin widen so that as much heat as possible can transfer to the air. It helps if the air is cool so it can chill us down. A third cooling mechanism works manually: turning on the air conditioner.

No one with any sense exercises in high heat or high humidity. Humidity really throws the system off. Even on a perfectly balmy day, high humidity fills the air with water vapor. Thus, the air can't evaporate the sweat off your skin because it can't absorb any more moisture. The sweat drips off you instead of evaporating. Your body gets hotter and hotter. Your heart pumps faster and faster, trying to carry more and more hot blood to the skin to be cooled. You perspire more and more and lose so much water that your blood becomes too thick. Thicker blood makes your heart work harder and holds less oxygen so your organs and muscles become starved. You get hotter and hotter until you start cooking yourself to death.

You don't cure heat injuries. You prevent them. To this end, there are a few hard-and-fast rules.

**Exercise according to how hot it feels, not how hot the thermometer says it is.** Temperature isn't the only factor in how hot you feel. If there's no breeze, you feel hotter. If the day is bright and cloudless, you feel hotter. If you have a tail wind instead of a head wind, you feel hotter. And, of course, it's not the heat, it's the humidity. . . . So, whenever you want to know how hot it is, use our Sultry-Swelter Factor (see Table 4.1). You've heard of the wind-chill factor. Well, this is its hot-weather opposite number.

### TABLE 4.1
### SULTRY-SWELTER FACTOR

| | |
|---|---:|
| Air temperature | 75 degrees F. |
| + | |
| High humidity | 10 degrees |
| + | |
| Very bright, cloudless sky | 10 degrees |
| + | |
| No wind | 5 degrees |
| Total | 100 degrees F. |

Start with the air temperature. If the humidity is high, add ten degrees (twenty if the humidity is very high). If the day is bright and cloudless, add another ten to twenty degrees. If there's little or no wind, add another five to ten degrees. If there is a wind, but it's a tail wind, add five to ten degrees. Wind at your back doesn't cool you nearly as much as wind blowing in your face. (You could reverse your course, so the tail wind becomes a head wind. Then you don't have to add the five to ten degrees.)

Using these figures, then, a 75-degree day, calm, bright, and very humid, has a Sultry-Swelter Factor of 100 degrees—much too hot to be doing anything more strenuous than lying under a shady tree.

**Drink water.** Plain cold water is one of your main lines of defense against heat injury. Drink it in prodigious amounts throughout the day, then drink as much as you can hold plus a little more right before you do anything strenuous. Drink about a cup of water every fifteen minutes during your exercise and drink until you feel cooled and refreshed after you've finished exercising. Don't wait until you feel thirsty. By the time you're thirsty, you're already a quart or so down and in big trouble. Worse yet, some people on their way to heatstroke never do get thirsty. If you are bicycling, you may not feel as hot as, say, a runner will because the wind in your face evaporates your sweat. However, you're still sweating and you must replace that water.

Make that water cool or cold. It won't give you cramps, no matter what the old coaches' tales say. And you don't need anything fancier than water—no sodas, soft drinks, sugar water, or so-called sports drinks. All your body uses from any drink is the water, so why adulterate it? Adding sugar, salts, caffeine, alcohol, or whatever only slows down the absorption of the water. (Sugar, in fact, indirectly dehydrates you instead of replacing your fluids.) Those sports drinks or electrolyte replacement drinks have odd balances of minerals—how do you know that's what your body needs?—and are often high in sodium and low in potassium and zinc. If you're worried that you've sweated so abundantly that you've lost vital minerals, drink a glass of orange juice after your exercise and eat a few pieces of dried fruit.

**Dress lightly.** Wear as little clothing as decently possible. The more skin you have exposed, the more surface area is cooled by breezes and evaporation. Wear 100 percent cotton, because cotton breathes and lets the moisture pass through.

Wear a vented or mesh hat to keep the heat of the sun off your scalp. If you wish, put a wet handkerchief on your head or the back of your neck. You can buy hats that have pockets in which to insert frozen gel packets that stay cold for more than an hour.

**Don't take salt tablets.** You probably get more than enough salt in your diet already, and the tablets, indirectly, draw water out of your system.

**Don't drink alcoholic beverages.** They lower your heat tolerance and dehydrate you.

**Do everything you can to stay out of the heat.** Exercise in the air-conditioned splendor of your rumpus room or some local health spa or gym, or exercise in the cool of the early morning or the late evening (if that's safe).

**Slow down.** For every five degrees above seventy degrees Fahrenheit, take about 5 or 10 percent longer to finish your exercise. If the heat's getting to you, cut short your exercise for the day.

# Taking the Chill Out of Cold Weather

There's nothing like exercising on a crisp, cold day. Picture it: fresh snow, sparkling sunlight, clear air. You're dressed in layers so you're snug when you walk out the door. As you start moving, your body cranks out its own heat and you peel off a scarf or a sweater so you're never too warm or too cold. You're invigorated. You and the world are aglow. No way will you ever be that refreshed in hot weather: you can warm yourself up in cold weather but you can't cool yourself off in warm.

It's true that cold weather rarely comes off as such a picture-book fairy tale. Often, the streets are dangerously icy, the winds viciously cutting, the wind-chill factor low enough to freeze off your nose. You have to have enough sense to know when it's too cold.

This is where the wind-chill factor comes in. Wind cools you by evaporating the moisture from your skin. Thus, you feel cooler at twenty-five degrees with a ten-mile-per-hour wind blowing than at twenty-five degrees with no wind. In fact, twenty-five degrees with a ten-mile-per-hour wind feels like ten degrees.

# TABLE 4.2
## WIND-CHILL FACTOR: EFFECTIVE TEMPERATURE ON EXPOSED FLESH*

*Air Temperature (Degrees Fahrenheit)*

| WIND SPEED (MPH) | 45 | 40 | 35 | 30 | 25 | 20 | 15 | 10 | 5 | 0 | −5 | −10 | −15 | −20 | −25 | −30 | −35 | −40 |
|---|---|---|---|---|---|---|---|---|---|---|---|---|---|---|---|---|---|---|
| 5  | 43 | 37 | 32 | 27 | 22 | 16 | 11 | 6 | 0 | −5 | −10 | −15 | −21 | −26 | −31 | −36 | −42 | −47 |
| 10 | 34 | 28 | 22 | 16 | 10 | 3 | −3 | −9 | −15 | −22 | −27 | −34 | −40 | −46 | −52 | −58 | −64 | −71 |
| 15 | 29 | 23 | 16 | 9 | 2 | −5 | −11 | −18 | −25 | −31 | −38 | −45 | −51 | −58 | −65 | −72 | −78 | −85 |
| 20 | 26 | 19 | 12 | 4 | −3 | −10 | −17 | −24 | −31 | −39 | −46 | −53 | −60 | −67 | −74 | −81 | −88 | −95 |
| 25 | 23 | 16 | 8 | 1 | −7 | −15 | −22 | −29 | −36 | −44 | −51 | −59 | −66 | −74 | −81 | −88 | −96 | |
| 30 | 21 | 13 | 6 | −2 | −10 | −18 | −25 | −33 | −41 | −49 | −56 | −64 | −71 | −79 | −86 | −93 | −97 | |
| 35 | 20 | 12 | 4 | −4 | −12 | −20 | −27 | −35 | −43 | −52 | −58 | −67 | −74 | −82 | −89 | −97 | | |
| 40† | 19 | 11 | 3 | −5 | −13 | −21 | −29 | −37 | −45 | −53 | −60 | −69 | −76 | −84 | −92 | | | |

WIND CHILL

Exposed flesh may freeze in one minute

Exposed flesh may freeze in thirty seconds

†Wind speeds above 40 mph have little additional chilling effect.
*Adapted from a table prepared by the National Oceanic and Atmospheric Administration.

That subjective ten degrees is called the wind-chill factor (see Table 4.2). When you figure out your wind-chill factor, add in any wind you create while moving. If, for example, you are riding a bicycle at ten miles per hour, add that to the atmospheric wind (say, ten miles per hour). Thus, if you're riding on a perfectly acceptable twenty-five-degree day, but the combined wind is twenty miles per hour, your wind-chill factor is minus three degrees. And that's pretty darn cold.

We recommend that you stay indoors if the wind-chill factor falls in the warmer end of the light gray zone of our chart. We insist you stay indoors if it falls in the colder end or anywhere in dark gray zone. Only Paul Bunyan could withstand cold like that.

## FROSTBITE

If all you do is normal daily exercise about town, you probably won't come near either of the two kinds of cold injury. The first and less serious, frostbite, actually freezes your skin. Basically, your body reduces the circulation to your skin in order to keep your interior warm. Ice crystals form in your cells just as they do in a frozen steak. It starts with cold, white, firm patches, usually on your nose, cheeks, ears, fingers, or toes. There's no pain. If it continues, the frozen area starts to tingle or sting. Finally, the frozen area turns gray and numb. Again, there's no pain because the cold has damaged your nerves. If you do get a mild case of frostbite—a very few small white patches on your nose, cheeks, ears, fingers, or toes—go back indoors and rewarm the areas by soaking in a warm, not hot, bath. If you have anything more serious than that, see a doctor. Never rub or massage frostbitten patches with your hands or with snow, because you'll push the sharp corners of the ice crystals through the cell walls and permanently damage your skin.

## HYPOTHERMIA

The second type of cold injury, hypothermia, can be deadly. Hypothermia means an abnormally low internal body or core temperature (95 degrees Fahrenheit or under). Your body's first loyalty is to the core, where all the important machinery resides. When you're very cold, your body concentrates its heat in the core. The blood vessels near your skin narrow to reduce heat loss. This makes your skin pale. Your hands and feet get cold. If your core temperature continues to fall, your muscles tense up to manufacture heat. Those muscle contractions make you shiver. If you don't warm up, your heart beats more and more weakly and irregularly and finally stops altogether.

As with heatstroke, some people are more susceptible than others, but we all become more prone to hypothermia as we enter our sixties and seventies. The same drugs that may provoke heatstroke also make you vulnerable to hypothermia. Also, smokers take note: nicotine slows your circulation. The absolute rule here is: if the day feels cold, it *is* cold. It doesn't matter if someone else is warm. If you feel cold, you're cold.

You don't have to have frostbite to die from hypothermia. If your clothes are wet, either from rain, snow, a dunking in the river, or copious sweating, and you're caught in a brisk wind, you can become dangerously chilled in forty- or fifty-degree temperatures. The 1,500 victims of the sinking of the Titanic didn't drown—they were all wearing buoyant life jackets. They died from hypothermia.

If you are shivering uncontrollably, your speech is slurred, and/or your hands and feet feel clumsy, you have the early stages of hypothermia. Get inside immediately and rewarm yourself in a body-temperature (not hot) bath. Then put on dry clothes, snuggle under some blankets, and treat yourself to warm soup or cocoa. If you've gone beyond shivering, your skin is pale blue or pinkish blue (and perhaps a bit puffy), and/or your coordination is bad, you've got a moderate case of hypothermia. Get home immediately and follow the instructions for mild hypothermia. You may, however, advance to the middle stages because you can't get home soon enough. In this case, take off your clothes and bundle up in blankets or a sleeping bag. Sip warm nonalcoholic liquids. (Alcoholic beverages actually increase heat loss.) See a doctor as soon as possible. If you get to the serious stages of hypothermia, you'll be in no condition to do anything for yourself. Just pray that someone gets you to a doctor immediately.

The key to preventing hypothermia is to stay warm and dry.

**Dress in layers** using the wind-chill factor, not the temperature, as your guide. Depending on the weather, wear two to four layers.

The underwear layer works to get rid of perspiration. If you don't perspire very much, silk T-shirts and long johns may be the most wonderful thing you've ever put next to your skin: they're loose, sensuously smooth, unaggressively warm, and yet they don't show under your clothes or make your over-clothes feel tight. Cotton is also nice, although it tends to fit like last year's skin and make you feel like an overstuffed sausage as soon as you don your second layer. The problem with silk and cotton is that they absorb all of your body moisture and get cold and clammy when you sweat.

If you do perspire, wear underclothes that carry the perspiration away from your skin. This action is called wicking, and it's a buzzword of the mid-1980s. The current favorite materials are polypropylene and other plastics that don't absorb water. The drops of water wick immediately to the surface of the cloth. Polypro and its friends dry quickly so you dry quickly. However, they too feel like you're wearing sausage casing.

Wool also wicks but differently. The wool fibers themselves absorb water droplets and water vapor. Thus, wool wicks the moisture away from your skin so you feel dry, although the outer surface of the wool stays wet. Wool has a drawback: it's itchy.

Bicyclists, take note. Polypro dries quickly by evaporation. Evaporation cools your skin. Wool dries slowly but keeps its warmth when wet (it's the only fabric that can do that). Therefore, wool doesn't cool your skin. It follows, then, that if you wear polypro on a cold winter's ride, the wind is going to chill you to the bone unless you wear a breathable windproof shell as your outer layer (see below).

After the underwear, add layers depending on the wind-chill factor. Your middle layers work to trap a layer of warm air around you while still letting moisture evaporate. Wool and cotton knit shirts and sweaters work well, as do pile-lined pants. You might want to put on a sweater over that. Then a natural or synthetic fleece, pile, or down jacket. There are several new dense synthetic insulators on the market. They keep you warmer with less bulk than down or other parka insulators so you don't have that roly-poly look. Polyester fleece and polyester fibers also insulate extremely well.

You need an outer layer not to warm you but to protect you against wind, rain, or snow. If it's windy, wear a light wind shell over everything else to block the freezing gusts. We prefer shells made of breathable, seam-sealed synthetics woven with hundreds of thousands of microscopic pores so that perspiration can escape. If it's not gusty, a parka or jacket can double as a shell.

If it's raining or snowing, you'll need a waterproof coat and rainpants. Again, we recommend those seam-sealed breathable fabrics. Nonporous plastic and rubber rain gear are nothing more than portable steam baths. You may be protected from the rain, but you're sopping wet inside from your own sweat.

There's nothing colder than wet feet. Waterproof your shoes with a silicone seal made especially for shoes, or buy a pair of waterproof boots that breathe and are light and comfortable for long walks or runs. (Ha! If you find such a perfect animal, please write us and tell us what and where.)

On icy roads, wear waterproofed shoes with studded waffle treads. If you can't find shoes or boots already waffled and studded, resole an old pair of shoes with these grips. Ask your running-shoe store or deal direct by mail. Or, if you don't like walking on studded snow tires, try spiked rubbers. Pull these black rubbers over your shoes, and let the sharp metal teeth tear into the slickest ice. They are, however, weird and uncomfortable to balance on. No matter what, carry a metal-tipped cross-country ski pole for stability on the ice.

Don't forget your hat. You lose at least 30 percent of your body heat through your uncovered head because the blood vessels in your scalp don't constrict in the cold the way the vessels in the rest of your body do. (If you get too hot after exercising for a while, take off your hat first and you'll vent off 30 percent of your heat.)

Cover every other exposed bit of skin, if necessary, wearing gloves, scarves over your nose and mouth and around your neck. (If you wheeze in cold weather, wear a surgical mask over your mouth and nose to warm the air before you inhale it. They are cheap and available in most large drugstores and surgical supply houses.) Choose your socks the way you chose your underwear. If your feet are usually cold, wear silk or polypro liners underneath your thick wool socks. Or wear a pair of thin wool socks under a pair of medium or thick wool socks. Make sure that the bulky socks don't make your shoes too tight or your feet will get numb and frostbitten from poor circulation.

If the weather is extremely cold, we advise you not to

exercise in it. If you insist, you might want to try a trick that some runners and cross-country skiers in Minnesota use: Before you put on any clothing, rub on a thin layer of petroleum jelly. Then pile on all your garments. The grease will feel uncomfortable, but it will add a valuable layer of insulation. (Men, take note: be sure to rub the petroleum jelly over *every* part of your body. Frostbite is no respecter of privacy.)

**Drink plenty of water.** The cold and the heavy breathing during exercise draw moisture out of your system, indirectly reducing the amount of oxygen feeding your muscles and organs.

**Forget about bicycling** unless the roads are thoroughly cleared of snow, ice, slush, and salty-sandy sludge. The salt will eat up your tires and everything else will trip you up. Ride an indoor bicycle instead or take up a wheelless sport.

# Preventing Sun Damage

Whether we're talking bright summer days, sunbathing at the beach with the glorious sun bouncing off sand and water, or clear winter days on the ski slopes, the sun's rays can damage your eyes and burn your skin.

## PROTECTIVE SUNGLASSES

Ordinary sunglasses ease the glare so you don't squint, but they may in fact be more dangerous than walking around bare-eyed. When you wear sunglasses, your eyes relax and your pupils open wide to let in all those harmful ultraviolet (UV) rays. This could lead to sunburned eyes now and to cataracts down the line.

Solution: buy sunglasses with specially treated lenses. The tag on the glasses will tell you what percentage of UV rays are blocked. Aim for 99 percent. Some opticians can coat your existing sunglasses with a compound that also cuts out almost 100 percent of the ultraviolet rays.

## SUNSCREENS

Considering that the incidence of all types of skin cancers has mushroomed, it makes no sense to sunbathe, exercise, or even work in the garden without wearing a sunscreen with a Sun Protection Factor (SPF) of 8 or higher. The FDA requires every tanning lotion or cream to list its SPF. The SPF tells you how much longer it will take you to burn with the screen than without. With an SPF of 8, for example, it will take you eight times as long to burn as it would without the screen. If it usually takes you half an hour to burn at the beach, it will take you four hours with an SPF 8 screen. You will tan, but much more slowly. The most effective sunscreens contain PABA (para-aminobenzoic acid). People allergic to sulfa drugs may also be allergic to PABA. There are a few sunscreens without PABA. Check the labels. Also, fortifying the sunscreen with 2 to 5 percent vitamin E appears to reduce even further the damage from ultraviolet rays.

Plain oils and other nonscreen lotions and creams don't prevent burning, no matter what your friends tell you.

When you walk, run, cycle, swim, row, canoe, or kayak outdoors, you become attuned to the weather. You watch the weather news on television, and you remember what tomorrow's relative humidity is supposed to be. You feel the seasons come and go, and you revel in the clean air after a summer storm or the first snowfall. This is a joy, not a burden—an extra little gift you get from exercising that you might otherwise have missed entirely.

# Eating to Win and Lose—Weight, That Is

"**D**on't go swimming for an hour after you've eaten or you'll get cramps and drown." That's probably the most popular superstition about food and sports, but there are others, equally wrong. "Don't drink water during a workout or you'll get cramps," for instance. Or, "take salt tablets if you exercise in hot weather." Or, "protein builds muscle."

Nutrition is a book—or fifty books—in itself. All we can do in *Going the Distance* is to condense two lifetimes of research and experience into a few brief pages of guidelines.

Should you eat before you exercise? The answer, basically, is yes, if you wish; no, if you don't feel like it. There are no hard-and-fast rules. If you skip a meal or snack and you feel weak or fuzzy-headed partway through your constitutional, eat something next time. If, one day, you try eating before your workout and it leaves you feeling logy, don't eat as much next time.

The old rule was: don't eat for two hours before you exercise or you'll get the runs or stitches in your side (from gas). Essentially, that's the origin of the superstition about swimming on a full stomach. The theory was that when you're digesting food, much of your blood supply is diverted to your digestive tract and away from your muscles. Insufficient blood to the muscles, it's true, might cause a mild cramp in a leg or arm. If the blood does go into your exercising muscles instead of your digestive tract, you may be surprised by some indigestion.

Don't worry about this rule. Many dedicated runners, swimmers, and cyclists eat all day. If they waited until their stomachs were empty before they exercised, they'd never get on the road. Your chance of cramps and indigestion are exceedingly small as long as you don't eat a *heavy* meal within one hour of exercising.

Some people find they must eat or at least snack before and during any vigorous exercise or they run out of energy. Certainly, long exercise sessions—a two- or three-hour bike ride, for example, or a half-day row across a lake—demand some sort of nourishment along the way. Common sense dictates that the more demanding the exercise, the lighter your immediate pre-workout food should be. Usually, you feel too ponderous to exercise after a heavy meal, but you may be an exception.

What should you eat before exercise? As a general rule, starchy snacks give you more quick energy than protein or fatty foods. First of all, they digest much faster. Second, the body can convert starches and sugars into energy easily. Some people enjoy cookies, candies, or soft drinks immediately before or during a workout. However, as a general rule, sugary snacks give you a quick boost and then, five or ten minutes later, plunge you into greater fatigue than before.

Whether or not you eat before or during your exercise, drink water—lots of water—before you start working out, and more every twenty minutes thereafter in hot weather. Water is your first and main line of defense against heat and cold injuries. (See Chapter 4 for a full explanation.) Don't take salt tablets in hot weather. Even people on low-salt diets eat enough salt to prevent heat injury. Salt tablets require huge amounts of water to dissolve and process them, so you wind up with a net water loss. Worse yet, extra salt in your cells makes your heart work harder in hot weather than it otherwise has to.

# Tips for Good Nutrition:
# The 20:20:60 Diet

The concept of a balanced diet has changed over our lifetimes. In the fifties, Miss Monahan, our sixth-grade teacher (wasn't she yours?), taught us to balance every meal by eating one serving from each of the Four Basic Food Groups—meat/eggs; milk; vegetables; bread. Later, nutritionists preached the Seven Basic Food Groups, and then promoted an elaborate system of Exchange Groups of one sort or another.

Now, they've streamlined the concepts down to three categories—protein, fats, and carbohydrates—with a small nod to vitamins and minerals. We've simplified this system even further into our 20:20:60 Diet.

The 20:20:60 Diet tells you what proportion of your food each day should be protein, fat, and carbohydrate. These proportions appear to follow the dietary balance nature intended for us. That means we run less risk of many of the major diseases of our generation, including digestive and breast cancers, heart disease, high blood pressure, kidney trouble, arthritis, and adult-onset diabetes.

The 20:20:60 Diet allows you the glorious freedom to eat whatever appeals to you, within reason. As long as you eat the proper amount of protein, for example, you can make that protein a sizzling piece of juicy steak, or a scoop of cottage cheese.

The 20:20:60 Diet, combined with two to four hours per week of one of the aerobic exercises in Parts Two and Three, lets you lose weight gradually, if you're so inclined, without feeling deprived or toying around the edges of malnutrition. While you still have to restrict your calories somewhat—modern science has yet to invent The Pig-Out Diet for Instant Weight Loss—the 20:20:60 Diet is a lot easier on the psyche than all the fad diets ever invented.

The 20:20:60 rules are simplicity themselves.

## BALANCE YOUR DIET BY PORTIONS

The idea is to assign a percentage of your diet to each of the three categories. Basically, meat should total no more than 20 percent of your daily calories; fat should total 20 to 30 percent; carbohydrates should fill up the rest of your calories.

This means, of course, that you have to know how many calories you should eat each day. That varies with height, size of frame, and (especially) ideal body weight. Most people have a pretty good idea of what they should weigh. That's as good as any figure to use for your ideal weight. (Don't figure your calories based on your current weight if you're overfat. The excess fat on your frame doesn't burn calories and so doesn't figure into the equation.)

You need anywhere from 12 to 15 calories per day per pound of ideal weight. Choose 12 calories per pound if you have a small frame or want to lose weight. Choose 15 calories if you have a large frame and are six feet or over in height. For example, if your ideal weight is 110 and you want to lose weight, you'd multiply 110 pounds by 12 calories per pound, for a total of about 1,320 calories a day. If your ideal weight is 170 pounds, you're fairly tall, and you don't want to lose weight, you'd multiply 170 by 14 calories for a daily allowance of about 2,380 calories.

## AVOID EATING TOO MUCH PROTEIN

Miss Monahan told us that large helpings of protein—meaning meat, with side orders of eggs or cheese—guaranteed strong, healthy bodies. Ah, how the times have changed. Now, while we acknowledge that we need protein to maintain and repair the cells in our bodies, we have learned that too much protein causes more diseases in the developed countries of the world than too little protein does—ills such as various cancers, heart disease, kidney trouble, osteoporosis (too much protein draws calcium out of your bones), and more.

Miss Monahan quoted the old adage that protein builds muscle and told us about football training tables, groaning with steaks and hamburgers. While it is true that protein builds muscle, 20 percent of your daily calories is plenty. In fact, most people can get along with 15 percent very healthily. Poor Miss Monahan. She'd never recognize today's training tables, loaded with bowls of pasta and loaves of whole wheat bread.

To estimate how much protein you should eat, figure that your 20 percent means anywhere from three to six three-ounce portions of lean beef, chicken, or fish or the equivalent in beans, nuts, or other vegetarian protein-laden foods, depending on your size. You don't have to be terribly precise—you aren't measuring reagents for a chemistry class.

Meat, eggs, and cheese are high-fat foods. That's one reason why eating large amounts of red meat is associated with high blood LDL cholesterol levels. Vegetarians and fish eaters have the lowest LDL levels.

It looks like chicken offers some protection against accumulating LDL in the bloodstream because chicken fat is monounsaturated, a type of oil that appears to clean the cholesterol out of the bloodstream. The same is true for the polyunsaturated fat in fish, especially cold-water fish.

## CUT DOWN ON FAT BUT DON'T CUT IT OUT

Fat is also crucial to survival—it is the heart's favorite fuel and helps build nerves and cell walls. It also carries oxygen to all body tissues. Excess fat, however, clogs up our arteries.

Your fat allowance can be anywhere from 20 to 30 percent of your total daily calories. If you want to lose weight and/or your doctor has told you to cut back on fat, aim at 20 percent. For a small person, 20 to 30 percent fat equals a total of 2½ to 3½ tablespoons of oil, butter, meat fat, and any other dietary fat per day. For a large person, 20 to 30 percent fat equals 4 to 6 tablespoons of the same. Otherwise go as high as 30 if you like. Don't drop below 20 percent, because your heart needs fat for fuel, and you don't want to set off irregular heartbeats.

To calculate roughly how much fat you're eating, figure a tablespoon of butter or oil contains about 100 calories. (Don't forget there's also fat in most meat and in cookies, cakes, candies, and pies.) Most of your fat allowance should come from oils.

*Polyunsaturated fats* include corn, soy, cottonseed, safflower, sunflower, sesame, walnut, and wheat-germ oils. They lower total blood cholesterol levels—the good HDL as well as the bad LDL. Let polyunsaturates total about half of the fat in your diet.

*Monounsaturated fats* include olive oil, chicken fat, peanut oil, and mustard-seed oil. They lower blood LDL cholesterol but leave the good HDL cholesterol alone. They should total about one half of the fat in your diet. (However, go easy on the peanut oil until researchers determine whether eating too much of it damages human arteries.)

*Saturated fats* include butter, lard, vegetable shortening, fat on meat, and coconut and palm oil, often used in processed foods. They raise bad cholesterol levels in the bloodstream. Eat them sparingly.

We think you're better off avoiding margarines, which are polyunsaturated oils solidified by a process called hydrogenation. Thus, they no longer are completely polyunsaturated, and they no longer confer the health benefits of the oil in its original form. There is also some evidence that they may be carcinogenic (cancer-causing). Cook with oils, and, if your health permits, give yourself a treat once in a while of real butter on your toast or potato. But ask your doctor first.

## LOAD UP ON HEALTH-GIVING CARBOHYDRATES

Nutritionists urge us to eat more fruits, vegetables, whole grains, nuts, and beans. These carbohydrates are rich in starches, sugars, and fibers. Carbohydrates are our bodies' most important fuel. In fact, our brains and nerve cells use nothing else. The body also uses carbohydrates to form many of its sub-protein building blocks (called amino acids). We even need carbohydrates in order to burn fat for energy.

No one rails against eating too much carbohydrate, although nutritionists do warn against simple carbohydrates, meaning sugar, and against refined or white flour. (Don't panic. We figure we're all entitled to a few chocolate chip cookies as long as we also eat lots of whole grain cereals and fresh, raw fruits and vegetables.) Nutritionists also complain that we eat too few complex carbohydrates (meaning starches and fibers) and therefore come down with myriad digestive difficulties and, it appears, various kinds of cancers of the digestive tract. In addition, if we don't supply our bodies with enough carbohydrate, our bodies literally consume themselves, burning muscle tissue in order to save for our brains what little carbohydrate there is.

For people who exercise, carbohydrates stand second only to water in importance in the diet. They supply energy for our exercising muscles and help our body strip fat off our hips and bellies and burn it as fuel. If we don't eat enough complex carbohydrate, we quickly run out of steam.

You don't have to count or measure carbohydrates. Use them to fill up the rest of your calorie allowance after you've allotted yourself 20 percent protein and 20 to 30 percent fat.

Try to make *at least* half of your carbohydrate intake complex carbohydrates. This will give you the fiber and vitamins you need as well as keep you from gaining weight. Do allow yourself a jelly doughnut once in a while, though, or you'll feel so deprived, you won't be able to stay on this—or any other—diet.

## CONSIDER VITAMIN AND MINERAL SUPPLEMENTS CAREFULLY

At first glance, it may appear that the 20:20:60 Diet doesn't concern itself with vitamins and minerals. Not to worry. They come with the territory. If you make 60 percent of your diet whole grains, beans, nuts, and fresh raw fruit and raw or lightly cooked fresh vegetables, you'll wind up eating an abundance of B vitamins as well as vitamins A, C, D, E, some iron, calcium, magnesium, potassium, and just about all of the trace minerals.

Still, we all wonder at one time or another whether we need vitamin and/or mineral supplements. We can't answer that for you because we don't know the state of your health, or what you eat each day, or whether you're allergic to any of the ingredients used in vitamin and mineral pills. We ourselves take moderate doses of supplements, always with meals to make sure they're fully absorbed. We have been known to skip an occasional meal, or to eat hot fudge sundaes for lunch instead of fruit salads, and we want the insurance those little pills give. We don't believe in huge doses of supplements. Our bodies don't know what to do with such overdoses, and some can be thoroughly toxic. We consider the following amounts of supplements to be reasonable:

- 1,000 milligrams of *calcium carbonate* from oyster shells to keep our cells functioning properly, help our muscles contract, maintain cell membranes, aid the blood to clot, and prevent osteoporosis. Insufficient amounts of calcium (or magnesium) may lead to muscle cramps. The National Institutes of Health say postmenopausal women need between 1,200 and 1,500 milligrams a day to prevent osteoporosis. (We make sure the labels on our bottles read 1,000 milligrams of *elemental* calcium. That says how much actual calcium we're swallowing. It is possible for a 500-milligram calcium pill to contain only 100 milligrams of calcium.) We need magnesium and vitamin D to absorb calcium.

- 700 milligrams of *magnesium*—to balance the calcium. We need magnesium so our bodies can manufacture proteins, keep our muscle fibers working properly, conduct nerve impulses, and help convert carbohydrates into fuel.
- 2,000 milligrams of *vitamin C.* We need vitamin C to help our bodies absorb iron, B vitamins, and vitamins A and E. We also need it to keep our immune systems functioning and to produce various hormones and connective tissues. We take plain old ascorbic acid (in the form of calcium ascorbate powder mixed into orange juice) because it is cheap and is as effective as any health food compound. (Note: Some doctors say we should take no more than 1,000 milligrams a day or we risk diarrhea or, worse, kidney stones. We, along with many researchers, believe the risk of either problem is extremely small. We also think that 1,000 milligrams is not enough to help us absorb sufficient iron or to prevent bladder infections. Still, to be on the safe side, we recommend increasing the dose gradually by, say, 250 milligrams every few weeks. If, at any point along the way, you develop diarrhea, drop back 250 or 500 milligrams and stay there. And if you know you're prone to kidney stones, take only 1,000 milligrams of vitamin C.)
- We differ on our *iron* intake. Sandra takes 80 milligrams a day. This is about four times the U.S. Recommended Dietary Allowance, but there's good evidence that the RDA for iron is set too low, especially for menstruating women, so we recommend the 80 milligrams—but only for menstruating women. Ron takes 20 milligrams. Men and postmenopausal women need one-quarter to one-half the iron menstruating women need. Everyone needs iron to manufacture red blood cells, which carry oxygen throughout our bodies. Too much iron, however, damages the liver, kidneys, and heart. Vitamin C makes the iron more absorbable.
- 6 milligrams of *vitamins $B_1$* and *$B_2$.*
- 9 milligrams of *vitamin $B_6$.*
- 18 micrograms of *vitamin $B_{12}$.*

- 40 milligrams of *niacin,* another B vitamin.
- 1 milligram of *folic acid,* another B vitamin.

We need the various B vitamins to power the digestion and conversion of carbohydrates and fats into energy and, in the case of folic acid and vitamin $B_{12}$, for manufacturing new red blood cells.

- No pantothenic acid, biotin, choline, inositol, or several other B vitamins. We get plenty from meat, nuts, and raw vegetables.
- No vitamins A or D. We get enough A from vegetables and the cold-water fish we eat, and our bodies manufacture plenty of D every time we go out in the sun. When we tried supplements, our skin got dry and itchy.
- No vitamin E. There's no proof for any of the claims that it makes you live longer or prevents wrinkles. Besides, we get plenty of vitamin E from whole grains and nuts.

If you decide to change your diet, do it gradually. Don't give up everything you love in a single morning; you'll be miserable. Make small changes—more vegetables for lunch or fruit for dessert after dinner. They'll probably lead to other changes down the road.

Your new exercise program will help, because many people just naturally start eating more healthfully after they start to exercise regularly. They just don't feel like eating fast-food hamburgers anymore; instead, they crave salads and fresh fruit. As long as you exercise, everything else will come along in its own time.

# Arthritis, Asthma, Back Pain, Depression, and the Rest... Rx: Exercise

**Y**ou may be reading this chapter because you've just been diagnosed as having high blood pressure, diabetes, asthma, arthritis, or osteoporosis. Or perhaps you're in the midst of menopause, or grappling with low back pain or depression. You've already talked to your doctor about your condition and asked all the questions you could think of. You wondered whether you should exercise at all, and your doctor has okayed—in fact, encouraged—exercise. You're reading this to find out how to go about exercising in your condition. You're about to discover that exercising is the most effective and most pleasant way to conquer any of these problems.

Forty years ago, when a doctor told a thirty-five-year-old woman that she had high blood pressure, he prescribed complete bed rest—for life. Today, he'd prescribe exercise.

Twenty years ago, when a doctor treated a fifty-year-old man suffering from the pain and stiffness of osteoarthritis, she advised a rocking chair and a good book. Today, she'd advise exercise.

Ten years ago, when a doctor counseled a wheezing, breathless forty-five-year-old woman with asthma, he told her to stay away from all vigorous activity. Today, he'd recommend exercise.

Today, exercise strikes most of us as a commonsense approach to overcoming many of our physical and emotional ills, and medical research has confirmed our intuition. Recent studies have shown that exercise often beats any drug in controlling and sometimes curing the ills that creep up on us in our middle years—high blood pressure, asthma and allergies, arthritis, back pain, osteoporosis, diabetes, menstrual difficulties, menopause, depression, and anxiety.

Even after your doctor approves an exercise program, it may take courage to get yourself moving. It's all very well for a doctor to tell a woman with asthma that she should exercise and that it may even help her to breathe easier. But this woman is bound to fear she will be one of the many asthmatics who get sicker, not healthier, from exercising. All her doctor's reassurances to the contrary, she must collect her courage to jump in for her first swim. Or, take the man whose knees ache and throb at the slightest movement. How does he force himself to get up from the couch and take a walk?

It helps to remember that moving around will actually make you feel better over the long haul. But, most of all, you must feel confident that you are doing the right sort of exercise the right—and safe—way for your condition. That's what this chapter is all about.

Note: We have not included any information here on heart disease. It's true that exercise is one of the most important prescriptions doctors give cardiac patients. However, heart disease is beyond the scope of this book; anyone with heart or coronary artery disease should be under a doctor's supervision.

In fact, if you have any chronic or acute illness, whether it is mentioned in this chapter or not, you should ask your doctor whether it is okay for you to exercise and, if so, how to do it. This book is no substitute for your doctor's advice.

# Arthritis

(Note: If you have low back pain, turn to that section later in this chapter.)

Seventy-five million Americans suffer occasionally and

mildly from some kind of arthritis. Twenty-two million have moderate arthritic problems and three million must endure severe cases. One out of every ten patients walks into a doctor's office complaining of arthritis.

Most people with arthritis think they've got some incurable disease they can't do anything about. They're mistaken. Very few people are crippled by arthritis. Most have only minor pain and even then will go weeks or months between flare-ups. Most can get rid of their pain and make their bodies move smoothly and easily. And exercise is their most important ally, their greatest painkiller.

Technically, arthritis is an inflammation of the joints. By this definition, an arthritic joint is red, warm, swollen, and tender when squeezed. However, many arthritis specialists use a looser definition: any painful condition of the bones, joints, or muscles.

The most common arthritises all respond extremely well to exercise:

- *Osteoarthritis*—by far the most common form since we all get it if we live long enough.
- *The strain-and-pain localized insults* such as Achilles tendinitis, sprained ankle, metatarsalgia, and swimmer's shoulder, all discussed in detail in Parts II and III.
- *Fibrositis,* a disease formerly described as "all in your head" but now recognized in medical texts as a real though puzzling arthritic phenomenon. In fact, exercise is just about the only therapy for fibrositis.

The milder forms of *rheumatoid arthritis* also respond to exercise, but since this disease requires constant medical care, it is beyond the scope of this book, as are the rest of the more than 100 kinds of arthritis. Either they must be treated by powerful prescription drugs or they are extremely rare or quite serious.

You've probably heard that arthritis comes from wear and tear, meaning that arthritis develops if you use a joint too much. Fortunately, this is more myth than fact. Runners—even those in their sixties, seventies, and eighties—who run long distances on concrete (not the most hospitable surface to run on) don't show any more arthritis than nonrunners. Likewise, people who operate pneumatic drills for twenty or thirty years don't show any more arthritis than people who don't put such stress on their joints. In fact, no studies have ever proved a connection between overusing a joint and developing osteoarthritis.

A few people do develop osteoarthritis from repeatedly abusing a joint—pitcher Sandy Koufax's arthritic elbow and basketball star Willis Reed's arthritic knees come to mind—but, even among professional athletes, this is rare. No one knows why one person develops wear-and-tear arthritis and another doesn't.

Generally, it works the other way around. You are more likely to develop osteoarthritis from a sedentary life than an active one. Activity lubricates your joints and keeps them pliable. That same lubricating effect prevents pain and flare-ups if you already have osteoarthritis. Daily exercise, in fact, is just about your only hope for keeping your arthritis under control (unless you've got severe knee or hip problems that require replacement surgery).

The most common arthritises—the ones that respond so well to exercise—all share the following features:

- Pain in one or only a few sites
- Joints may or may not be warm, swollen, or tender
- No morning stiffness
- No fever
- Typical pain sites: end finger joints, hips, knees, neck, lower back, elbow, shoulder, ankle, ball of foot, hand, wrist.

If you suffer a flare-up of one of these arthritises, we recommend trying home treatment for a few weeks before you consult a doctor. If you have none of the warning symptoms listed in the following section, and if the pain is bearable, you can't hurt yourself by waiting. If you do go to the doctor, chances are you'll be sent home with a prescription for self-care anyway.

## WHEN TO SEE YOUR DOCTOR

As a general rule, you don't have to see a doctor as soon as your joints start hurting. Arthritic complications usually occur slowly. However, certain symptoms are signals to see a doctor immediately:

- If you have a fever, especially if it's over 100 degrees Fahrenheit, you probably have an infection or a severe type of arthritis.
- If you have swelling or severe pain in just one or two joints, you may have gout (one of the arthritises not covered in this chapter), an infection, or another of the more urgent forms of arthritis. (Arthritis in one or two joints is, oddly, more serious than arthritis in several joints.)
- If you have intense pain or excruciating tenderness, you may have gout or one of the other arthritises that require prescription drugs to control.
- If you can't use the affected joint, you may have broken a bone or otherwise injured it and need immediate medical care to prevent permanent stiffness.
- Likewise, if your pain comes from an injury, you may have broken something.
- If you have back pain that runs down the leg to the foot, or if your hands or fingers tingle or are numb, or if an area of your head is numb when you move your neck, you may have nerve damage, an extreme emergency.

See your doctor immediately if you have any of these symptoms. In addition, if you have none of these symptoms but your problem has lasted for longer than six weeks, see your doctor.

The odds are better than twenty to one that you'll have none of the above symptoms. Instead, you'll have the usual, less threatening sorts that go away slowly over several weeks. In this case, modern medicine can do little for you. When the pain is acute, rest the aching parts of your body, apply a warm compress or a heating pad if it helps, and, perhaps, take two aspirin tablets four times a day. Unless the pain is severe, don't mask it with pain-killing drugs because you may then use the inflamed joint and injure it further.

## HOME TREATMENT FOR ARTHRITIS

Rest the affected body part. Take the pressure off of it by elevating it whenever possible, carrying it in a sling, or wearing a brace, and avoid anything that makes it hurt. (You'll find braces and splints at hospital supply stores and well-equipped drugstores.) If you don't have any swelling, and heat feels good, apply warm (not hot) compresses or a heating pad or sit in a warm bath. If you do have swelling, and cold doesn't hurt, apply cold compresses for ten minutes every few hours during the first day or so. Time is the drug of choice here, but a couple of aspirin four times a day are okay, though they probably won't help much. Stay away from painkillers because they kid you into believing your ache is gone, so you're likely to go out and reinjure yourself. If you're overweight and your pain is in a weight-bearing joint such as hip or knee, you're overtaxing those areas. Try to get down to a reasonable weight to slow down the damage.

No matter what type of minor arthritis you get or where it hurts, you need gentle exercise in order to heal properly. The idea is to back off the offending movement until the pain has subsided. In the meantime, do gentle stretching and toning exercises to move the joint through its entire range so it doesn't stiffen up. Exercise is your only hope for a healthy, fully functioning joint.

Exercise makes your bones stronger by drawing calcium into the bone cells. Exercise strengthens your muscles. These stronger muscles support and stabilize the joints. Tendons and ligaments become stronger and more pliable the more they're used, and they, too, stabilize and support your joints. Cartilage becomes healthier as well. Cartilage has no blood supply, so the only way it gets nourishment and oxygen and cleanses itself of wastes is through movement. Therefore, if your cartilage is deteriorating, as it does in osteoarthritis, exercise is your only hope for preserving what you have and making it stronger.

When a flare-up is severe, don't do anything to aggravate your already sore tissues. Keep your movements gentle and undemanding, but be sure to move your joints through their entire range of motion every day to prevent permanent stiffness. When the pain is not severe, do unjarring, regular exercise—walking, cycling, or swimming, indoors or out, or any of the other aerobic exercises described in Parts Two and Three, *as long as they're comfortable.* Don't do anything that puts pressure on an affected joint or jerks or overstretches it. These exercises not only kill pain and revitalize joints but also prevent further flare-ups. Arthritis proves the use-it-or-lose-it adage. If you don't use your body, it will decay out from under you, joint by joint. If you use it, the odds are you will be able to move freely and without pain for the rest of your life.

# Asthma and Allergies

Three percent of the American population have asthma. Ninety percent of asthmatics are likely to have an attack when they exercise, at least under certain conditions. Twelve percent of the population have some sort of allergic disease, and of these, about 30 percent will have asthma attacks when they exercise, even if they don't have such bronchial spasms at any other time. In addition, another 3 or 4 percent of the population have no allergies and never suffer from asthma except when they exercise. Doctors once believed that exercise-induced asthma was different from "true" asthma. They've since decided that asthma is asthma, no matter what the trigger may be.

The word *asthma* describes heavy or difficult breathing caused by certain chemicals in the throat that build up enough to trigger a spasm (contraction) of the smooth muscles around the small air tubes (bronchi) in the lungs. During the spasm, the tissues in the bronchi swell and produce sticky mucus that plugs up the airways.

In a mild asthma attack, more precisely called a bronchospasm, you cough, breathe rapidly, or can't catch your breath; you wheeze, especially when you exhale; and your chest feels tight or aches or you get a stitch in your side. Your throat hurts and your head aches. You may even have a stomachache. For the five to fifteen minutes the typical attack lasts, you feel as if you're drowning—you're perfectly conscious and yet you can't do a thing about it. The entirely understandable panic is as much a part of asthma as the wheezing, but it probably makes the spasm worse. Most of these attacks disappear quickly if they're handled properly. In serious episodes, you also sweat and become flushed or pale or turn blue. (Note: These symptoms are also the signs of some types of heart disease. If you've never had an asthmatic attack before and one suddenly comes upon you—especially if it hurts rather than aches when you breathe—see your doctor immediately.)

Asthma is hard to pigeonhole. It's not a disease. It's not caused by a germ or a poison. Quite often, but not always, an asthma attack is triggered by an allergic reaction. People with asthma aren't sick. They simply suffer occasional bronchial spasms. Still, fear of those occasional spasms may dominate their lives, and one of the things they fear most is exercise.

## EXERCISE FOR ASTHMATICS

It's true that exercising too strenuously or breathing cold or dry air may set off an attack. However, many asthmatic athletes have found ways of exercising without triggering a spasm. In fact, in the 1984 Olympics, 67 of the 597 competitors had exercise-induced bronchospasms. Of them, 41 won medals in sports ranging from basketball and cycling through swimming and water polo.

If you have a history of asthma and you exercise regularly, you are likely to suffer fewer attacks and your attacks will probably be less severe. Also, exercise opens your bronchial passages wider than when you're sedentary. (Most of this effect comes during the first two minutes of exercise.) However, you *must* consult with your doctor first before setting out on any exercise program. Your doctor might recommend an electronically monitored exercise stress test to see how well you tolerate exercise and how hard you can work before an attack occurs.

You have several strategies to prevent exercise-induced spasms. Since cold or dry air may set off an attack, warm the air you breathe, especially in cold weather, by wearing a surgical mask, a mouthless ski mask, or a scarf over your nose and mouth. Breathe only through your nose to warm and humidify the air before it gets down into your throat. Or swim, play water polo, kayak, canoe, or row—the air just above water is naturally warm and moist. (However, some asthmatics are sensitive to the nitrogen chloride gas given off by swimming pools. These people should try to work out in outdoor pools, where the chlorine can dissipate, or in fresh or salt water.) If pollen or dust sets off the spasm, wear a surgical mask or some other nose and mouth covering that filters out small airborne particles.

Researchers have confirmed what many asthmatics have discovered on their own: the more strenuous the exercise, the more likely an asthma attack. Therefore, keep your exercise at a very moderate pace and warm up for twenty minutes instead of the usual five or ten minutes to whittle away the spasm-inducing chemicals in your throat. Walking and cycling are popular dry-land sports for asthmatics. Running is often too strenuous. Cross-country skiing works for asthmatics if they figure out how to keep the air warm and moist enough—masks are usually enough, but not always. Indoor exercise works very well for those asthmatics sensitive to cold, pollens, and dust.

Exercise in short bouts, say less than six minutes, and then stop and rest or move around very gently for two or three minutes; repeat this pattern several times during your workout. Since your air passages open wider during the first two minutes of exercise, this on-again, off-again technique opens those passages again and again.

If you require medication to control asthma, your doctor will probably prescribe a drug to be inhaled about fifteen minutes before exercise. Cromalyn and other powdered or aerosol inhalants should prevent any attacks during exercise, but your doctor can also give you a drug to carry with you just in case. The inhalants and aerosol forms of these drugs have few side effects for active people. The oral form may cause tremors or shakiness.

Some people simply cannot do any sort of exercise without going into spasm. However, most asthmatics can indeed exercise if they choose the right sort and take adequate precautions. In other words, if you want a full and active life, the odds are that your asthma won't get in your way.

# Depression and Anxiety

Exercise chases away the blues and the worries. After about three weeks of regular aerobic exercise of the sort we describe in this book, people with mild to moderate depression or anxiety will notice they've climbed at least partway out of the pit. For people with severe depression, anxiety, or phobias, exercise is at least as effective over the short haul as psychotherapy. (Because one of the symptoms of severe depression is the inability to face even the simplest tasks, severely depressed people usually need someone to encourage them to get out of the house and into their walking shoes.)

When you are depressed or anxious, the blood flow to your

brain decreases. Exercise increases blood flow to the brain and so reverses the effects of depression. Also, when you're depressed, your brain produces various hormones and other chemicals (including catecholamines and indoleamines). British researchers have found that a mere ten minutes of exercise three times a week releases various chemicals, including norepinephrine, which neutralizes those depression chemicals, and serotonin, which is a mood-elevating chemical produced inside the brain.

In most of the research projects about the effects of exercise on emotional illness, running was the sport tested. However, in our experience, all of the other aerobic sports described in Parts Two and Three work as well as running to break the chains of depression and anxiety.

# Diabetes

About ten million Americans have diabetes, and 600,000 more develop it each year, an increase of about 6 percent annually. As we Americans get older, fatter, and more sedentary, our chance of coming down with diabetes increases to about one in five by age seventy. (Some doctors say they expect every plump patient over the age of seventy to show symptoms of diabetes.) By the year 1990, the number of diabetic Americans will have doubled to about twenty million.

## TYPE I AND TYPE II

There are two types of diabetes, both involving how sugar gets from the diet into the cells of the body, but the mechanisms are so different that some doctors consider them to be two separate diseases.

In adult-onset (also called non-insulin-dependent or Type II) diabetes, the most common form, your body provides the chemical ways to use sugar but the cells don't respond properly. Ninety-five percent of American diabetics have this form of the disease. Eighty percent of these people are over forty, and most adult-onset diabetics are overweight. Most of them can control their diabetes and escape the long-term dangers of heart and kidney disease simply by watching their diets and doing aerobic exercise.

In juvenile-onset (also called insulin-dependent or Type I) diabetes, the body doesn't have the chemical apparatus to process sugar in the first place. Five percent of American diabetics have this type, which must be treated with insulin and which, without adequate care, may lead to blindness, heart disease, gangrene, kidney failure, and death. However, it too may be controlled by diet and exercise in conjunction with insulin.

Every cell in the body uses sugar to fuel at least some of its work. In a normal system, sugars from food enter the bloodstream, where they travel to each cell. When the body senses there is sugar to process, the pancreas releases insulin to help the cells absorb the sugar. Each cell draws its portion of sugar out of the blood and uses it for energy.

In a diabetic, the system breaks down in one of two ways. In the Type I, insulin-dependent diabetic, the pancreas doesn't produce insulin, so the cells are deprived of the chemical key they need to unlock the door and let sugar in. Type II, non-insulin-dependent diabetics have plenty of insulin. In fact, they may produce too much. But for some reason their bodies are resistant to insulin, and, again, they can't draw sugar out of the bloodstream and into the cells. Either way, the cells become starved. The excess sugar floating around the bloodstream damages the blood vessels. As the blood passes through the kidneys, the kidneys siphon off the sugar, and a lot of water, into the urine. If not controlled, all of this leads eventually to eye damage, gangrene, kidney disease, heart disease, stroke, diabetic coma, even death. Unless Type II diabetes is carefully controlled, it is as dangerous as Type I.

The causes of Type I diabetes are still a mystery, but doctors believe that heredity and viral damage both play a part. Because it is an extremely serious medical problem, diabetics must work in very close association with their doctors. Once the blood sugar is under control, doctors usually recommend the types of aerobic exercise described in Parts II and III, because exercise has been known to reduce a diabetic's insulin requirements. However, a Type I diabetic exercise program is beyond the scope of this book because it involves so many complicated factors, including precautions against sudden drops in blood sugar and possible diabetic coma.

Type II diabetes runs in families. In addition, some racial and ethnic groups (such as blacks, Hispanics, and American Indians) are more susceptible, although it's possible that these groups have a higher incidence than the general population because they tend to be heavier and more sedentary. Obesity is probably the deciding factor in Type II diabetes. As a fat cell becomes more and more stuffed, it gets fewer and fewer receptors for insulin and, as a result, more and more hitches in processing sugar. The chance of getting Type II diabetes doubles for every twenty pounds of fat gained—especially, oddly enough, for women whose fat is mostly above the waist. (No one yet has come up with a thorough explanation of why fat above the waist is statistically associated with Type II diabetes.)

The symptoms of Type II diabetes are so mild and appear so gradually that often neither patient nor doctor notices them until a chance blood test sets off alarm bells. If there are obvious symptoms, they may be some or all of the following: excessive thirst or hunger, frequent urination, rapid and unexplained weight loss, drowsiness, itching, unhealable skin infections, blurred vision, tingling or numbness in the feet (due to poor circulation in the legs).

## EXERCISE FOR DIABETICS

Once Type II diabetics have had thorough medical workups and have followed doctors' orders—by taking medication, if necessary; by following the correct high-fiber, low-fat, high-complex-carbohydrate diet; and by bringing their blood sugar under control—they will, no doubt, be told to exercise. It is important that their blood sugar be brought down first. Otherwise, exercise may raise blood sugar instead of lowering it.

(This is a relatively new regimen for Type II diabetics. Many years ago, diabetics were put on low-carbohydrate diets and told not to exercise. The low-carbohydrate diets kept diabetics almost at a starvation level, and if they tried to exercise, they'd burn their own protein—that is, muscle—and fat for fuel.)

The aerobic exercises described in Parts Two and Three are the wonder drugs of the diabetes circuit—with the exception of running and skipping rope for those with very serious diabetes or foot trouble. First of all, exercise helps everyone lose weight, and weight loss is the first defense against diabetes. In addition, sustained exercise (that means regular aerobic exercise following the rules in Chapter 3) also makes your muscle cells more sensitive and responsive to insulin and thus lowers your need for insulin medication. It teaches your muscles to require less insulin to pull sugar out of your bloodstream. Also, it helps use up the sugar in your bloodstream so it can't stay around to damage blood vessels. It makes you less hungry, a real boon if you have always felt hungry on your diabetic diet. It also helps you get rid of stress and tension. This is important because stress often sends your blood sugar out of control. Exercise also lessens the ability of blood-clotting platelets to clog up the arteries the way they do when blood sugar is high. And, of course, it reduces your risk of heart attacks and lowers your blood cholesterol.

Exercise does have one complication, however: it makes you more responsive to insulin. Therefore, as you exercise during the first few weeks, you have to figure out how to adjust by taking less insulin or eating more. Don't exercise on an empty stomach or when your insulin medication is reaching its peak effect. Eat during exercise if necessary or eat extra complex carbohydrates right before exercising. If you inject insulin, don't inject it into the part of your body you're exercising. You don't want your exercise to plunge your blood sugar to below-normal levels. Also, if you have serious diabetes, your circulation is impaired, especially in the feet and legs, and you're more likely to develop infections from the slightest rash, cut, or blister on your foot. And, because of your poor circulation, you're more likely to suffer heatstroke or hypothermia. Be extra attentive to all the precautions listed in Chapter 4. (Also, in cold weather, you use more energy just to stay warm, so adjust your diet and insulin accordingly.) Be sure to consult with your doctor about these questions.

# High Blood Pressure

Hypertension, or high blood pressure, is one of the most prevalent serious diseases in the United States, afflicting sixty million Americans. What makes hypertension insidious is that it has no outward symptoms. You don't feel sick when your blood pressure is too high. In fact, some people feel better with high rather than normal blood pressure. But if the pressure isn't brought down to a normal range, the heart works harder and harder, becomes weakened and damaged, and in the process damages the kidneys and arteries. Such destruction builds over the years. Then, one week you might notice that you're terribly winded after walking up three stairs. Or your ankles might swell and you might show signs of kidney inflammation or kidney failure. Or perhaps you suffer a stroke or heart attack.

Now you understand why almost every time you visit the doctor, someone takes your blood pressure. That inflated cuff around your arm measures the pressure of the blood against the artery walls. This pressure results from several factors, among them how much blood flows through your arteries, how strong each heartbeat is, and how elastic your artery walls are.

Blood pressure is reported as a fraction. The upper, larger number, called the systolic phase, measures the pressure or force your heart exerts to push the blood through your arteries each time it contracts, or pumps. The lower, smaller number, called the diastolic phase, represents the pressure in your elastic artery walls when the heart is filling with blood between beats.

Normal blood pressure is said to be about $120/80$, but it is the diastolic (lower) number that's most important. Anything over 90 diastolic is considered high and warrants medical care. If you have high systolic (upper number) pressure—say, a little more than 100 plus your age—your doctor will do further checkups, but usually high systolic over a normal diastolic reflects something temporary happening in your circulation and isn't serious. (Blood pressure lower than the normal figures isn't harmful unless it is a symptom of some underlying disease or is the result of injury, shock, or loss of blood.)

## EXERCISE FOR HYPERTENSIVES

If you have any significant degree of hypertension, your doctor will probably forbid you to exercise until your blood pressure comes down to near normal. The explanation is simple: When you exercise, your systolic pressure goes up. If your systolic pressure is already high, your heart must work so hard, it could give out. Once your blood pressure is under control, your doctor may well advise moderate leg exercise, such as walking or cycling, for they have been shown to lower high blood pressure. Running is probably too strenuous for most formerly sedentary hypertensives. And most experts warn against arm exercises such as rowing and cross-country skiing unless your blood pressure is very well controlled, because arm exercise makes more demands on the heart than leg exercise. Swimming comes in as a definite maybe. It's an arm exercise, but one that uses legs as well in a balanced fashioned, spreading the strain throughout the body. Also, swimming's horizontal position is much easier on the heart, so it's fine for most people. As hypertensives get into better shape, their doctor may okay rowing and cross-country skiing, too.

Any sort of weight lifting—whether the official sort with barbells or resistance machines, or the unofficial sort such as moving couches or shoveling snow—is off-limits for hypertensives. These sorts of exercise spike your blood pressure to dangerous heights. Stay away from them.

# Low Back Pain

One out of every two human beings suffers pain in the lower part of the back at times—the price we pay for erect posture. Low back pain is more likely to strike the overweight or sedentary or the person who exercises only sporadically, but none of us is immune. When you're barely enduring an excruciating backache, it doesn't help to recall that just about everyone develops back trouble at one time or another and that modern medicine can't do a thing for you. It's just you, your back, and time, working this thing through together.

Most back pain comes from minor injuries, usually during some motion in which your lower body moves forward while your upper body abruptly arches backward. Sometimes, however, you don't remember hurting your back at all. In terms of diagnosis, it really doesn't matter—whatever the cause, neither you nor your doctor will be able to tell exactly which of the hundreds of ligaments, muscles, and joints were first injured. Once you hurt a small area of your back, your body immobilizes it (the way a plaster cast immobilizes a broken bone) to give it time to heal. It immobilizes the injury by sending the surrounding muscles of your back into piercing, gnawing, wrenching spasms.

The back is a complex instrument whose core is the spine, a stack of bones (the vertebrae) connected by short ligaments. The ligaments cross the disks. There is a disk between each vertebra to act as a shock absorber, to cushion the spine, and to permit it to curve and bend smoothly. Other, long ligaments run up and down the spine. Muscles attach each vertebra to the one above or below it, and other muscles connect each vertebra to the one two away, three away, and so on. There are also small joints between each vertebra, and these joints are connected by ligaments and lubricated by sacs of slippery synovial fluid.

Most back problems involve these ligaments, muscles, and joints. If the gelatinous material in the center of the intervertebral disks bulges out (herniates), that material may press on spinal nerves, causing great pain and serious damage, sometimes in areas far from the back. This is most likely to happen to people in their thirties and forties. The older you get, the smaller your chances of an acute herniated disk. In overweight people, small ruptures of fat into the back tissues may also cause low back pain. Minor disk protrusions act like minor low back problems and may be treated the same way. Serious disk problems involving rubbing on nerve roots are medical problems beyond the scope of this book.

## SYMPTOMS AND TREATMENT
## OF BACK SPRAIN

A back injury is a sprain, similar to an ankle sprain except for the back's own contribution, the muscle spasm. You have overstrained or wrenched a joint. Like any sprain, the area hurts and swells and may even bruise during the first twenty-four hours. The pain is usually most extreme in the inwardly curved part of the lower back. It may extend down into the buttocks.

In a sprain, the pain shouldn't go below the knee, and neither of your legs should be numb or weak. These are symptoms of a herniated disk and nerve damage. So are the following: pain is worse at rest or at night; difficulty urinating or moving your bowels; pain is worse when you cough or sneeze. If you have these symptoms, or if you are running a fever, the pain is severe, or if you hurt your back by falling hard, see a doctor immediately. If your back pain is moderate but is a new occurrence, you might want to consult your doctor anyway, just to play it safe.

That first day, you probably won't want to do anything but find a comfortable position and not move from it. Try lying on the floor or on a firm mattress with or without a bed board. Or try tucking a small pillow under the curve of your back to support it. Or try lying on your side in a fetal position, your knees tucked up toward your chest. This is also the way to get up off a bed or couch: tuck your knees up toward your chest, roll over onto your side, then sit up.

It's okay to take aspirin, which won't help too much, or other painkillers, as long as you don't get up and move around as if your back were healthy. Although some doctors prescribe muscle relaxers because they relieve some of the pain, we suggest avoiding these drugs. As painful as that spasm is, it is your body's way of protecting your back from further injury and giving it time to heal. If you can bear the pain, go along with your body on this one.

Cold compresses for ten minutes every few hours during the first day may decrease the pain and swelling. Don't apply heat for at least three days, if at all. (Most people say heat doesn't help much anyway.)

The pain will continue to be severe for the next two or three days. Continue doing whatever worked the first day. The pain, if you're lucky, will subside a little during the next week and become only nagging after that.

After that first week, or whenever you can honestly say you feel a lot better, try these gentle exercises. You need flexibility in your back to move easily without pain, and you need strong back, buttocks, and abdominal muscles to maintain good posture and avoid straining your back.

**Pelvic tilt:** Lie on your back on the floor with your knees bent and your feet flat on the floor. Tighten your buttocks and pull in your abdominal muscles so that the hollow of your back flattens against the floor (see Figure 6.1). This tilts your pubic

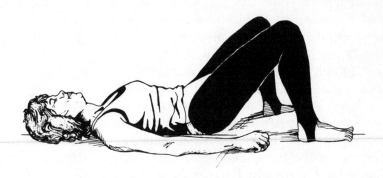

FIGURE 6.1 PELVIC TILT.

bone up. Hold for three seconds, relax, then repeat. Do three or four repetitions the first few days. Gradually, as you get stronger, work yourself up to twenty a day, done lying down, standing, or sitting.

**Sit-downs:** When your back pain is gone, do ten or twenty sit-downs every day to further strengthen your abdominal muscles for good solid back protection (see No-Stress Super Stretches in Chapter 3).

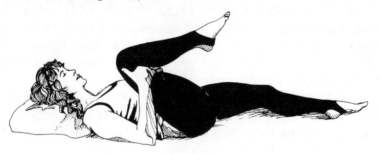

FIGURE 6.2  LOW BACK STRETCH.

**Low back stretch:** Lie on your back with a pillow under your head. Bring one knee up toward your chin, grab it with your hands, and hold it as close as possible to your body (see Figure 6.2). Exhale to curve your spine. Hold for three or four seconds, relax (and inhale), then repeat two or three times. Gradually work yourself up to twenty repetitions each day. When your back is better, graduate to the *back stretches* in the No-Stress Super Stretches, Chapter 3.

**Low back toner:** When your pain is better, strengthen your back muscles by sitting in a straight-backed chair or on the floor with your back against the wall. Push your shoulder blades into the chair back or wall (see Figure 6.3) and hold for five seconds. Relax. Repeat three times. Work yourself up to twenty repetitions a day. (You'll notice that your stomach muscles tighten as you push; this shows how much you use your abdominal muscles to support your back.)

It takes six to eight weeks for a back sprain to fully heal. However, many people reinjure their backs during the healing period, starting the cycle of pain all over again and further weakening the back for another and then another reinjury. That's one reason why back problems are so stubborn. If your back isn't well after six weeks, see your doctor.

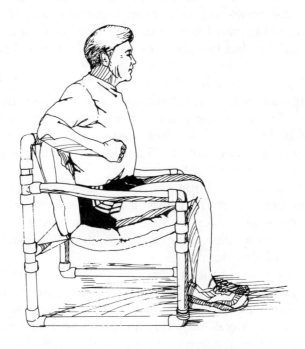

FIGURE 6.3  LOW BACK TONER.

## ONGOING EXERCISE PROGRAMS
## FOR THE BACK

Exercise—proper exercise—is the miracle cure for most low back pain. It helps regulate weight, produces natural pain-killers, and, most important, strengthens muscles. Strong, supple back muscles protect your back against sprains, while strong abdominals improve your posture and keep your back from swaying.

If you're uncertain about what exercises are good for your condition, ask your doctor or a physical therapist. In general, smooth and rhythmic sports, such as most of the aerobic activities in this book, work wonders. Walking strengthens the stomach and back muscles gently and gradually. Swimming is the back sufferer's favorite exercise because it tones every part of the body from an undemanding horizontal position. Some people with low back pain find the backstroke a miracle, others prefer the crawl, and still others can swim only if they wear something buoyant (such as an inner tube or float belt) around their middles, but just about everyone can swim. (See Chapter 14.)

Cycling is usually okay for people with back trouble as long as they ride upright instead of in the bent-over racer's crouch. The reclining posture used in recumbent bicycles is best of all, but recumbents are hard to find and more expensive than uprights. (See Chapter 7 for indoor cycling and Chapter 15 for outdoor cycling.)

Cross-country skiing helps most back sufferers because it is a smooth rather than jarring exercise that conditions the entire body. However, be sure not to bend over or overreach with your poles. (See Chapter 9 for indoor skiing and Chapter 16 for outdoor skiing.)

Rowing strengthens back and abdominal muscles quickly and most effectively and usually is kind to lower backs. However, some back sufferers cannot tolerate rowing. Whether you can canoe or kayak depends on whether it hurts when you round your back, as you inevitably will in these boats. Neither canoeing nor kayaking will strengthen your back and abdominal muscles as much as back sufferers need, but if you do sit-downs every day, you'll probably be okay. (See Chapter 8 for indoor rowing and Chapter 17 for outdoor rowing, kayaking, and canoeing.)

Running and skipping rope are too jarring for most back sufferers. Any forceful back-arching activity—back bends, lifting weights with a straight back, tennis, and golf, to name a few —are death on the back. Tennis forces you to make sudden shifts and strains in your upper body, and that's forbidden to people with back problems. But the worst part of tennis for your back is the overhead stroke, be it serve or smash, where you abruptly arch your back with all your might. Golf swings also push your back through abnormal arching, while you twist and thrust it as powerfully as you can through every kind of maneuver designed to sprain a whole string of spinal joints. Also on the forbidden list: twisting, touching your toes, and doing side bends.

But most back pain sufferers must exercise to ensure a healthy, pain-free future. It's up to you.

# Osteoporosis

Twenty-five percent of all women over fifty, and 15 percent of all men over fifty, are afflicted with osteoporosis. Several factors increase your chances for osteoporosis. Some are within your control; others aren't. If you are thin, and/or an alcoholic, and/or a smoker, and/or a Caucasian, and/or come from a family with a history of osteoporosis, and/or live a long life, you're at risk for osteoporosis.

When you have osteoporosis, your bones lose calcium, the mineral that makes them hard and heavy. Your bones become thin and soft yet brittle. The long bones of your arms and legs become shorter and weaker. Your vertebrae collapse in on themselves and you become shorter and hunched over. Eventually, your bones shatter at the slightest provocation: you step off a curb and your hip crumbles, or you open a window and your wrist fractures.

Statistically, osteoporosis strikes women earlier than men because men's bones are harder and thicker to begin with. On top of that, after menopause women lose much of their most effective ally in absorbing calcium: estrogen. Estrogen stimulates women's bones to absorb calcium from food. When estrogen levels drop, as they do during and after menopause, women absorb calcium much less efficiently.

The human body cannot perform without calcium. If your body does not receive enough calcium from the foods that you eat, it will steal the calcium from your bones in order to power your nerve and muscle cells and keep your cells intact. If that calcium isn't replaced, your bones cave in.

People over fifty must consume 1,000 to 1,500 milligrams of calcium a day in order to absorb enough to preserve their bones. For most people, this means taking a dietary supplement, because it's very hard to eat foods containing the necessary amount of calcium every day. Too much protein reduces the amount of calcium your body can absorb. Thus, moderate-protein diets prevent osteoporosis much more effectively than high-protein diets. (See Chapter 5 for more dietary information.)

## EXERCISE STRENGTHENS BONES

Your bones can't absorb all of this calcium if you don't exercise. Exercise is crucial in preventing and even reversing osteoporosis. When you eat enough calcium and then exercise, your muscles pull on your bones. Your bones respond by trying to toughen themselves by absorbing calcium. Each bone needs its own exercise. This means that to harden your leg bones, you must walk, row, cycle, cross-country ski, or row. To harden your arm bones, you must row, swim, cross-country ski, canoe or kayak, or walk carrying wrist weights. Running and cross-country skiing are dangerous for people with advanced osteoporosis because the danger of falling and breaking a bone is too great. Swimming hardens the arm and shoulder bones because you're pulling against the weight of the water, but it doesn't rebuild leg bones very well because your legs don't work against much resistance.

Outdoor exercise is better than indoor for fighting osteoporosis, because the sunshine stimulates your body to produce vitamin D, and you need vitamin D in order to absorb calcium efficiently.

If you think you have osteoporosis, consult your doctor about what sort of exercise is okay. People with advanced osteoporosis may not be able to do all of the sports in this book.

# Premenstrual, Menstrual, and Menopausal Symptoms

## EXERCISE MINIMIZES MONTHLY SYMPTOMS

Over the years, many women have told us that regular exercise throughout the month cuts down on the mood changes (depression, anxiety, and irritability) they used to experience before every menstrual period. Only recently, a few scientific studies have verified what experience has told us all along: women who exercise aerobically report that their premenstrual symptoms decrease significantly.

At first, we assumed we were seeing the same mood-altering effects seen in depressed and anxious people, and that's certainly part of it. But it's not the entire explanation, because women who exercise also tell us that their breasts aren't as tender, their feet and ankles don't swell as much, they don't feel as bloated or get as nauseated, and they don't get as severe headaches and backaches.

Exercise may lower the levels of estrogen in the system. Estrogen causes the body to hold onto salt, and salt causes the body to retain water. The water presses on the nerve tissue in the brain and spinal cord—thus the moods, headaches, and backaches. Water also causes swelling in various parts of the body, and intestinal upsets. Exercise drains off some of that water and salt in the form of sweat.

In addition, we're convinced endorphins are involved here. Endorphins are painkillers that the brain manufactures for itself throughout the day, but especially during exercise. They probably kill much of the discomfort premenstrual strain causes.

Although it's not the perfect cure, exercise also reduces or eliminates menstrual cramps, probably because it inhibits prostaglandins in the uterus. These powerful chemicals stimulate uterine contractions during menstruation and childbirth. And the endorphins produced during exercise mask the pain of cramps. Finally, regular exercise strengthens abdominal muscles, and stronger muscles are less likely to cramp up.

## EXERCISE AND MENOPAUSE

Very little research has been done on the effects of exercise on menopause, and the tiny bit that exists often contradicts women's personal experience. For example, no scientist has been able to prove that exercise diminishes the frequency or intensity of hot flashes, by far the most distressing symptom of menopause according to most women. Yet many women tell us that doing aerobic exercise almost every day has reduced, shortened, or weakened their hot flashes.

It's possible that exercise helps because it affects the hypothalamus. The hypothalamus is the region of the brain that controls emotions, body temperature, breathing (including breathing during a workout), and several other essential functions, including regulating the glands that, in turn, regulate the output of estrogen. The hypothalamus probably sets off hot flashes because it has become irritable and sends irregular spurts of hormones into the bloodstream. This raises the skin temperature anywhere from eight to twenty degrees. Exercise seems to calm the hypothalamus down again.

Many menopausal women complain they sleep only an hour or so at a time because they have frequent hot flashes during the night. With so little sleep, they become impatient and irritable, and that stress sets off more hot flashes, which cut into their sleep even more . . . and on and on. Aerobic exercise relaxes people and promotes deep, sound sleep. This is another way it interrupts the hot-flash cycle.

Read any list of the unpleasant side effects of menopause, and eventually you'll come to depression, anxiety, irritability, and anger. A good part of those mood changes come from lack of sleep, but some of them are due to lowered levels of norepinephrine, one of the chemicals that fight depression. Exercise increases the amount of norepinephrine and serotonin, the brain's own "happy pill."

Exercise is probably the most powerful medicine known today for these ordinary inconveniences of forty or more years of life. These aches and pains and chemical imbalances need more than drugs to set them right. They need a rebalancing that only exercise can provide. Even if you take drugs or require surgery, somewhere down the line, the doctor will tell you to exercise. Nature intended your body to be a perpetual motion machine. Truly it is written: use it or lose it.

# PART
# TWO

## Exercising Indoors

When most of us think about exercising at home, we think of Grandma's setting-up exercises, or the 98-pound weakling's barbells in the garage, or the high-kicking fitness star's workout on television.

Ah, but the five chapters in Part Two will show how home exercise holds riches far beyond flat midsections. The enormous rewards of genuine, whole-body aerobics await you in your living room. With a modest or moderate investment, you can walk, run, cycle, row, ski, or jump rope at home and get every bit as good an aerobic workout as anything you get outdoors. And the few of us with the wherewithal for a home pool can even swim at home. No commuting to a gym or bicycling trail. No traffic. No crowds. No prying eyes. No muggers. No snow, nor rain, nor heat, nor gloom of night. No inconvenience.

For most of us, home is the first place we think of when we decide it's time to get into shape. Exercising at home is enormously popular. Depending on whose statistics you believe, from 60 to 80 percent of us exercise at home, more than all the people who train or play in health spas and gyms and in the great outdoors combined.

Indoor aerobic sports do cost money—$10 to $20, at the low end, for a jump rope; $100 to $500 for a moderately priced exercise cycle, rowing machine, treadmill, or skiing apparatus. They also take up space. You have to have a place to set up your equipment and to store it when it's not in use—or, in the case of rope skipping, you've got to have room enough to swing the rope and not hit the ceiling or Aunt Minnie's Christmas vase. (Note: If you're short on space, look for folding rowers, exercise bikes, and ski machines.) Still, once you buy the equipment, it will last your lifetime, and you'll reap rewards in health a hundred times over.

Ambience is as important in an exercise room as it is in a restaurant. Working out in your garage may keep all of that clunky equipment out of the house, but it's dreary, lonely, dusty, and musty out there. It's cold in the winter and drab in the summer.

You'll enjoy your workout a lot more if the room is well lit, cool in summer and warm in winter, and roomy enough to exercise in comfortably. Give yourself enough room to add your own homemade diverting (and distracting) options to your equipment. Set a music stand beside the front wheel of your exercise bicycle, for example, so you can pedal and read a magazine at the same time. Or put your ski machine near the stereo so you can tune in your favorite music. Row and listen to Books on Tape through your pocket stereo's headphones. Watch the evening news; learn a foreign language from records or tapes; talk to friends on the phone; help your kids with their homework. Be creative and build variety into the game.

The following chapters are detailed enough to serve as short, practical introductory courses in each sport. Read through quickly to get a feel for each activity, then use the book as a how-to companion once you've made your choices. Whatever you choose, you'll be amazed to discover how much better you feel next month than you do now, and all you will have done is have a good time in the comfort of your own home.

# CHAPTER 7

# Exercise Bicycles: Pedal Power

**M**ention home exercise equipment and, nine times out of ten, the first thing most people think of is an exercise bicycle. These stationary bikes, also called ergometers (instruments that measure work or effort), have been around almost as long as rolling bikes and are far and away the most popular large piece of home gym equipment, and for good reason. They're almost sinfully easy to use —you don't need a single lesson to work one properly and you don't have to get used to it. Just climb on any time of the day or night, any weather, and pedal your way to strong legs and the same excellent aerobic workout that regular, outdoor bicycling provides.

Exercise bicycles make year-round fitness pals. They also make admirable training gizmos for outdoor cyclists when the weather turns nasty. "I don't feel I'm compromising anything when I ride my ergometer," says veteran cyclist James Wang, a sixty-year-old San Diego television producer. "If it's too hot or too wet, I get a perfectly good workout and get some reading done besides."

# The Pitch

Cycling indoors is almost as healthful as cycling outdoors. All you miss is the fresh air and sunshine. It strengthens your heart and lungs, gives you every aerobic reward promised in Chapters 1 and 2, and tones and firms all your hip and leg muscles. It doesn't do much for your upper body, but then neither does regular cycling. If you've got a good, solid exercycle and have adjusted the seat, pedals, and resistance properly, you're likely to pedal thousands of miles without a single injury. The ride is so stress-free that many doctors recommend indoor cycling for patients with many types of heart trouble.

**Don't ride an exerbike without a doctor's approval if you have chronic back or knee problems.**

# Buying and Testing Your Equipment

The enormous variety of exercise bicycles ranges from simple gadgets to hold your own bicycle immobile to computerized fantasies straight out of Buck Rogers. Middle-of-the-road exercisers, the most popular variety, indicate speed and distance and let you adjust the resistance on the pedals so you can feel as if you're riding uphill and downhill as you choose. High-tech ergometers provide electronic readouts of anything you need to know. They can even blow wind in your face.

Exercise bikes come in three basic—and quite different—types. Your choice depends on your budget, what feels comfortable, and whether you plan to use the machine as your primary form of exercise.

The *upright* model is probably what you picture when you think of a stationary bike. You sit tall in the saddle, with your hands straight out in front of you on fairly high handlebars. Usually, one large wheel turns at the front of the cycle as you pedal, although some models hide the mechanism inside a casing beneath the seat.

If you've gone shopping for exercise equipment lately, you've probably noticed that it's hard to find the familiar old-style exercise bikes, the ones that look like real bicycles. They still exist, and they're the most reasonably priced of exercise bikes, but they're fast being replaced by something that looks like a cross between Darth Vader's Go-Kart and a go-fast motorcycle. These high-tech models—renamed ergometers to make them sound more scientific—work just the way the old-fashioned ones do, but they have gadgets to tell you your speed, distance traveled, amount of resistance against the pedals, your pulse, blood pressure, lactic acid accumulation, oxygen uptake, whether you're in your target zone, the number of calories you've burned, and your performance compared to other people of your age, sex, and size. You pump the handlebars of some models up and down for upper-body exercise. Other models convert completely into rowing machines. A couple of models feature a fan propelled by the pedal shank. (To anyone who's sweated for an hour on an exercise bike, this sounds like a dream come true, but why not put a $20 fan in the room instead?) One $10,000 ergometer even comes with a video screen and tapes of outdoor scenes. The resistance on the pedals automatically increases as you ride uphill in your video and decreases as you coast downhill on the screen.

At this writing, prices for the utilitarian models start at around $150. Anything called an ergometer is likely to cost upwards of $250—with the decent models in the $600 range. One isokinetic pedaler (the term implies equal resistance throughout the pedal stroke) costs about $1,100. Many hospital supply rental companies and a few exercise equipment stores rent and lease exercise bicycles. However, the choice is usually limited to cheap, wobbly versions. Occasionally, a store will let you rent a cycle for a few months and then apply the rent you've paid to the purchase price.

The *recumbent* style works on the same principle as real, rolling recumbent bicycles (see Chapter 15). Instead of sitting up straight, you recline on a recumbent in a position similar to the one you take when reading in the bathtub. Recumbents are much more comfortable than uprights—they don't give you backaches or pain from ill-fitting seats—and they give a better aerobic workout and better conditioning for the legs and back. These machines are wonderful for exercise, and they're great for staying in training for outdoor recumbent riding. However, they won't train your legs for riding an outdoor upright because they condition your muscles to push forward from a slouched position instead of downward from a seated position. Only a few companies make recumbent ergometers (plain vanilla recumbents are even harder to find) and prices are a little higher than for comparable upright styles.

Test-ride your exerbike before you buy it. Be it upright or recumbent, the machine should feel very steady when you pedal *and* when you stand up on the pedals. If you feel the slightest wobble, try another brand. Pedaling action should be very smooth—reject any bike whose pedals seem to stick or suddenly speed up during any part of the stroke.

Any decent exerbike comes with adjustable resistance. Make sure the dial or handle is within easy reach from the seat. You are going to increase and decrease the tension while you're pedaling several times, sometimes within a single ride. Some manufacturers have hidden the adjustment gadget so you have to get off the bike—and sometimes even use a screwdriver—to tighten or loosen it. Perhaps they never rode one of their own bikes.

Make sure the bike is the right size for your body. The seat tilt *and* height should be easily adjustable, and if you or someone in your family is particularly tall, make sure the seat post (where the seat attaches) is extra long. When you sit on the seat, your leg should be slightly bent at the bottom of the pedaling stroke. When you pedal backwards, you shouldn't sway from side to side.

Get a firm seat that has no springs. You can always add a cushioned seat pad to make it easier on the tail bone, but you can't take the bounce out of a springy seat, and with a seat like that you'll waste a lot of your effort swinging from side to side as you pedal. (The same people who make seat and handlebar pads for outdoor bikes manufacture versions for exercise bikes. Our favorite brand provides a lot of cushioning with very little bulk, is machine washable, and seems to be indestructible. Many people favor sheepskin seat pads.) Keep the seat level or tilt it up a little at the front. This takes the strain off your wrists and arms.

Make sure your bike comes with toe clips or foot straps and be sure to use them. These devices will keep your feet from wobbling and sliding off the pedals and will permit you to pull up with one foot as you push down with the other. All this saves energy.

All but the simplest exercise bikes record revolutions per minute, speed, and distance. The revolutions per minute help you gauge how hard you're working, and the speedometer and odometer, while not essential, tell you how fast and how far you've gone. It's fun to know you've been riding at twenty miles an hour or that you've pedaled the equivalent of ten miles.

For safety's sake, if your bike has a wheel, make sure it's a solid one so that curious children can't catch their fingers in the whirling spokes.

The most useful accessory for an exercise bike is a book rack, made to attach to the bike itself, or a freestanding music stand placed in front of the bike. You can get an amazing amount of reading done while you pedal for forty-five minutes three or four days a week.

If you already own a bike, you might want to save money and turn it into an indoor exerciser with the third type of indoor exercycle: an accessory called a *wind trainer* or *wind-load simulator.* You attach your bike, usually but not always minus its front wheel, to this stand, and the fan or fans in the mechanism apply a drag to the rear wheel to simulate the way the wind pushes against you when you ride outdoors. This means you get a more demanding workout than from an upright or recumbent exerciser. These devices are wonderful for building leg strength and endurance, and they guarantee you a comfortable ride—as long as your bike is comfortable in the first place. Prices range between $70 and $150—quite a savings over stationary bikes and ergometers. Simulators are also portable and collapsible, to tuck away in a closet when not in use.

Buy the sturdiest wind trainer you can find. Most wind trainer frames flex during hard pedaling, but try for the most stable. Flexing wastes energy and sometimes stresses the forks of your bike (where the front wheel usually attaches). Wind trainers are noisy—not deafening, but noisy enough to send roommates out of the room. Put the trainer on a carpet to absorb some of the noise. Make sure your trainer fits your bike frame, or buy one that adjusts to various bike sizes. Almost all come in kit form, but some are easier to assemble than others. Choose one with a quick release lever for attaching and removing the bike (nuts take too much fussing). Look for Allen wrench fittings instead of nuts and bolts. They are easier to adjust. Look for a bottom bracket support that accommodates shift cables under the bottom bracket unless you're absolutely certain your shift cables won't get in the way. Finally, look for a noncorrosive finish—human sweat can eat away iron chains.

# Clothing

Dress in lighter-weight clothes than you would for riding outside. You're going to get quite warm. Pedaling in still air is oppressive. Aim a fan your way unless you're likely to get chilled. Drink plenty of water before you start riding, drink cool water during your ride, and drink plenty of cool water when you're done. Wear shoes to protect your toes and the soles of your feet.

# Warming Up

Start out with five minutes of easy pedaling on low tension to warm up your heart. Unless you're very stiff, you probably don't need to do stretching exercises before exercycling. Don't forget to cool down with another five to ten minutes of easy pedaling at low tension when you're finished.

# The Basics

### FIVE-MINUTE LESSON

Keep the tension low throughout your workout, especially as a beginner. You want to pedal for several minutes straight, and if you set the tension too high, your legs will give out long before your time is up. The first few days, you'll have to experiment. You want to be able to pedal at about 45 revolutions per minute and feel somewhat sweaty as you huff and puff your way into the aerobic zone. Adjust the tension up or down toward that goal.

Bicycles as a whole are so efficient that they do more than 30 percent of the work for you. Exerbikes are even more efficient because you don't have to push the wind away as you ride. Therefore, you may find yourself pedaling thirty miles an hour (according to your bike's speedometer) and still not be huffing and puffing. That's why you concentrate on tension rather than speed.

## SCHEDULE

As a beginner at exercise pedaling, ride as long as you can at low tension and moderate speed. As you get into better and better shape, you'll pick up speed and turn up the tension.

Your goal is to work up to seventy to ninety revolutions per minute at what feels like moderate tension. (In fact, you'll keep turning up the tension every few weeks, whenever the old setting feels too easy.) This workout should last anywhere from forty-five minutes to an hour, although thirty minutes is acceptable.

Once you can ride nonstop, follow this pattern for each workout: Warm up with five minutes of easy pedaling at low tension. Then, increase the tension until you're huffing and puffing aerobically. When you get your second wind and everything starts feeling a little easier, increase the tension a bit more to stay at that huffing-and-puffing level. When your time is up, cool down with a light-tension five-minute cruise.

If you're using a wind trainer, and you're a beginning cyclist, follow the same principles. Use easy gears instead of low-tension settings. If you're already a confirmed cyclist in good shape, warm up with five to ten minutes of easy pedaling (about ninety strokes per minute) in easy gears, moving slowly up into the higher gears. For the next fifteen to forty-five minutes, stay at the ninety revolutions per minute cadence but increase the gears until you're sweating and huffing and puffing. (See Beginner's Exercise Cycling Program on the following page.)

# Intermediate Exercise Cycling

You are an intermediate exercise cyclist if you can ride at a huffing-and-puffing aerobic point for forty-five minutes nonstop. If you want to increase your workout, add five minutes every other week and increase the tension a bit in the in-

## BEGINNER'S EXERCISE CYCLING PROGRAM

| WEEK | TENSION | REVOLUTIONS PER MINUTE | TOTAL MINUTES |
|------|---------|------------------------|---------------|
| 1 | lowest | 45 | 15 |
| 2 | lowest | 45 | 20 |
| 3 | lowest | 45 | 25 |
| 4 | lowest | 45 | 30 |
| 5 | lowest | 45 | 30 |
| 6 | lowest | 50 | 30 |
| 7 | lowest | 50 | 45 |
| 8 | lowest | 55 | 30 |
| 9 | lowest | 55 | 45 |
| 10 | lowest | 60 | 45 |
| 11 | lowest | 65 | 45 |
| 12 | lowest | 70 | 45 |
| 13 | a bit higher | 70 | 45 |
| 14 | same | 75 | 45 |
| 15 | a bit higher | 70 | 45 |
| 16 | same | 75 | 45 |
| 17–19 | same | add 5 each week | 45 |
| 20 | a bit higher | 90 | 45 |

Stay at the first week level until pedaling feels too easy, then increase the tension gradually and keep it there until, again, it feels too soft. You may also, if you like, add five minutes a week, every other week, to bring you up to one hour total pedaling time. Don't add minutes during weeks when you increase tension.

If this schedule moves too quickly for you, stay at each level for two or three weeks or until it becomes comfortable. If it goes too slowly, don't repeat weeks.

between weeks until you've worked yourself up to one hour nonstop.

## Masters Exercise Cycling

You are a master exercise cyclist when you can ride at a huffing-and-puffing aerobic point for one hour nonstop. To increase your workout, alternate between fast and moderate bursts of speed, and between high and moderate tension (to simulate up- and downhills).

If you're in particularly good shape, you might want to stick in several minutes of intervals—say, ride for thirty seconds as fast as you possibly can, then recover with easy pedaling in a moderate gear for a minute or two, then sprint again, and on and on, for perhaps ten minutes. Cool down for ten minutes the way you warmed up.

## First Aid

It's hard to hurt yourself on an exercise bike. If your back aches, tilt the nose of the seat up or down, or raise or lower the seat. If your hands get tingly or numb, tilt the nose of the seat up so that it takes the weight off your hands.

If you want to exercise indoors and can't figure out where to begin, start here with a stationary bike. You'll feel like an expert the moment you climb onto the seat, and you'll watch the miles pile up—say, 20 miles a day, five times a week, fifty-two weeks a year—5,200 miles a year, 520,000 miles in ten years—hundreds of thousands of miles and all you did was talk to your family or watch your favorite program on TV while you moved your legs around in large circles.

# Rowing Machines:
# Row, Row, Row Your Boat
# Gently Down the Rug

The sales of rowing machines have taken off in the last few years, and for good reason. Rowing is superb exercise for both upper and lower body and for overall health. It gives you more energy and a greater sense of confidence and well-being than any other indoor exercise we know except cross-country skiing. What's more, rowing machines are relatively inexpensive—good, workmanlike models start at $250—and they are small enough to stick in a closet or hide under a bed.

Don't be intimidated by the idea of rowing or you'll be missing one of the great joys of exercising. You don't need strong arms to row. On a rowing machine, as well as in a real rowboat with a sliding seat, your legs do more of the work than your arms.

## The Pitch

If you're looking for an aerobic exercise that you can do at home to strengthen your heart and lungs, burn calories, speed up your metabolism, improve your moods, give you more energy, and give you all the other payoffs you expect from exercise, rowing is it. Rowing does it all because you use all of your major muscle groups. (Exercycling and treadmill walking or running, in contrast, work only your leg muscles.) You strengthen and firm up your legs, buttocks, back, abdomen, and most of your upper body, developing longer, leaner, more graceful-looking muscles than most other sports give you.

With all of this, rowing movements are so smooth and gliding that there's no strain to the muscles or joints. You sit while you row, so there are no huge impact forces pounding away at your feet, legs, and hips. The rhythmic, regular movements of your oar strokes alternately relax and contract your muscles, so that many people who can't stand, walk, or run can sit and row. What's more, doctors now recommend rowing to cardiac patients and people with low back and disk problems. (The back question is tricky. Rowing helps some back problems but aggravates others. Ask your doctor.)

**Don't row without a doctor's approval if** you have severe back problems (e.g., advanced degenerative disk disease or spinal arthritis).

## Buying and Testing Your Equipment

Rowing machines come in two varieties. The first, most popular and least expensive, uses hydraulic cylinders—sort of like shock absorbers—to provide the resistance. You pull the two oarlike handles against the pressure from these pistons. The second, called a straight-pull machine, uses an electric motor with a braking mechanism or a flywheel braked by a fan or belt at the front of the machine for resistance. It has only one handle, which is attached to a chain, cord, or strap attached to the resistance mechanism.

Hydraulic machines are cheaper, more compact, and easier to store in your closet. Straight-pull machines cost more, but rowers prefer them because, despite the single handle, they feel more like real rowing. Although they place less of a load on the back and arms than hydraulic rowers do, straight-pull machines are noisy, bulky, and dangerous around children and pets. Both types come in simple models and fancier ergometers with readouts of speed, distance, calories burned, pulse, and just about anything else you can imagine. (The cheapest machines of all use metal springs or only one cylinder. Both arrangements are useless.)

Any rower should be very solid and stable. It shouldn't move, wobble, or jump as you row.

The stiffness or tension of the hydraulic cylinders should be easily adjustable. On some, you just move a knob up and down along the handle. This arrangement is convenient and alters the tension perfectly well, but it's imprecise. It is difficult to find the same spot on each oar to make both oars carry the same load. It is even harder to find your favorite spot again if someone else uses the machine and moves the knob. ("Infinitely adjustable" in the advertising copy is shorthand for "you'll never find the same spot twice.") We prefer rowers with notches or other easy-to-find settings. You'll need *at least five* settings. Ten are better.

As a general rule, the larger the diameter of the shock absorber, the sturdier the rower and the more even the rowing stroke. On the cheaper rowers, the load is uneven. That is to say, you don't feel enough effort at the beginning of the stroke but you feel much more somewhere in the middle. In effect, this cheats you out of any help from your legs because you use your legs most at the very beginning of the stroke. You wind up using your arms and shoulders all the way through the stroke. That's exhausting and could strain your back. The gas-assisted cylinders in the better rowers solve this problem because they keep the load even throughout the stroke. A good rower should move as smoothly when set on stiff tension as it does on a light load, and both oars should feel the same. On some cheap rowers, the cylinders are mismatched, so one arm works harder than the other.

On most hydraulic rowers, each handle moves in a single arc, starting down in front of you and then swinging up to a little past the vertical. This may be good exercise, but it isn't the way oars really move in the water. On some rowers, however, the oar handles are double-jointed, so you can feather them as if you're really rowing. This not only gives you a truer rowing motion but also exercises more muscle groups. It's not essential for your workout, but it's a nice touch and helps train you for real rowing on water. In any rower, the oars should move far enough forward for you to press your knees against your chest at the beginning of the stroke, and far enough backwards for you to stretch your legs straight and lean back slightly at the end of each pull. The oars should move smoothly, without getting hung up anywhere along their arc, and should be short enough or long enough for you to hold onto them comfortably.

All rowing machines use a sliding seat moving along a rail or track, the way real rowing shells do, so you can use your strong legs to help your weak arms push the oars. The seat should move freely, evenly, and relatively quietly, preferably on ball bearings or rollers along its track. Squeaks and strains are a sign of a weak frame or badly machined parts. We prefer rowers with tracks inclined downhill, like the pitched tracks in real racing shells, because they let you recover easily and more completely than level-track rowers after each stroke.

The seat should be on about the same level as the footplates, so that when you're all the way forward you sit in a kind of squat, with your shins almost vertical. This takes the load off your back and puts it onto your legs where it belongs. Some people prefer rowers with higher seats because they're easier to get on and off, but we're not sure that's as important as protecting your back.

The best seat is contoured to your bottom so you fit into the seat and don't slide around on it. A large and padded seat is second best, but padded certainly is better than uncomfortable. The seat should extend all the way to the back of the track at the end of your stroke, and all the way front, so that your knees are pressed against your chest at the beginning of the next stroke.

Make sure the footplates are arranged so that when the slide is all the way forward, your legs are bent and your shins are nearly vertical. Make sure your feet fit in the footplates. (The footplates are often too big for small people, too small for very big people.) The footrests should have a cup for your heel and should rotate or swivel as you push backwards during your stroke. The foot straps should adjust easily to hold your feet firmly in place and should rest on a comfortable place on your shoe without cutting or chafing.

Also, make sure your rower has a heavy, noncorrosible finish. You'd be surprised how quickly sweat eats away a cheap paint job.

Wearing exercise clothes, "test-drive" several models of rowers before you choose. You may have to try many different brands before you find one that fits. Fit is important because, unlike exerbikes, rowers are not adjustable (except for the oar tension). When you think you've found your dream machine, row on it for at least ten minutes. Work up a sweat. See how it feels when you try to find your rhythm. Feel for any little glitches or annoyances. Ask yourself whether you want to spend thirty to sixty minutes a day, year in and year out, on this machine.

With rowers, you get what you pay for. They start at $150, but for that price, you'll get something wobbly, with fixed footplates and perverse cylinders. Good quality, moderately priced machines run around $275. Middle-range, very functional machines retail around $350. The top-of-the-line, with almost every gadget imaginable, costs about $1,750.

# Clothing

Wear light hot-weather clothes when you row—you'll work up a good sweat. Be sure to wear shoes; otherwise the straps on the footplates will gouge large chunks of flesh out of the tops of your feet. You'll probably need a fan to cool you. Just don't get chilled. Drink plenty of water before, during, and after your workout.

# Warming Up

Warm up your heart by rowing slowly at the easiest tension setting for five to ten minutes. When you're done rowing for the day, cool down with the same lazy paddling for another five to ten minutes.

# The Basics

### FIVE-MINUTE LESSON

When you row on a rowing machine, you pull both oars together. The basic stroke is very simple. It's just a matter of

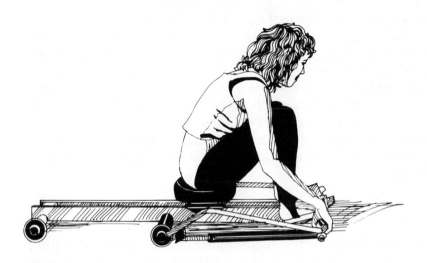

FIGURE 8.1  INDOOR ROWING (STARTING POSITION).

some simple coordination: pull with your arms and push with your legs.

Assume the starting position: With your feet strapped onto the footplates, grab onto the oar handles and move the seat all the way forward until your knees are bent and your thighs are pressed against your chest. Your back is slightly rounded. Your hands on the oar handles are down on either side of your ankles (see Figure 8.1).

Start pushing with your legs. They do most of the work at the beginning of the stroke. While keeping your arms straight, gradually straighten your legs. Your back is still slightly curved and your gaze rests about six feet in front of you. (Looking forward ensures good posture during the entire stroke.) As you straighten your legs, they carry your arms and the oars upward without much effort.

When your hands are just above your knees, start leaning back. When your legs are fully straightened (but not locked), pull the oars in to your chest or midsection (depending on your height). Don't lock your knees unless you're looking for knee injuries. Don't pull the oars past your stomach or chest unless you want backaches. Keep your back a bit curved, but lean back so your shoulders help with the pull. You should end up leaning back a little past upright (see Figure 8.2).

Begin your recovery by rounding your back slightly and stretching your arms forward until your hands (and the oar handles) move past your knees. Your legs are still straight. Now, slide your seat forward. (If your rower has a downhill track, gravity will do much of the work. If your track is level, you'll have to use your feet to pull against the foot straps.) Stop when you reach the starting position (knees bent, thighs pressed against your chest, oar handles down around your ankles).

## SCHEDULE

Start out slowly. Adjust the tension knob to the lowest setting and row only fast enough to warm up and get you gently huffing and puffing. If this feels like hard work, row for only a

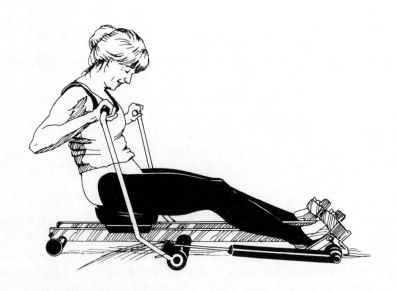

FIGURE 8.2  INDOOR ROWING.

minute, then rest for two minutes. As your condition improves, increase the amount of time you row and decrease the amount of time you rest. After a while, you'll be able to row for thirty minutes without stopping. Because rowing is such thorough full-body exercise, a half hour three or four times a week is probably enough to get you into shape and keep you there.

For aerobic fitness, you want to work steadily for thirty minutes at a low tension. Once you can row for thirty minutes nonstop (it could take you five months to reach this point), pick up your speed. Don't make the tension setting stiffer yet. High tension is too much effort to be aerobic. Count your strokes for ten seconds. In the beginning, you may be paddling only three strokes every ten seconds, or eighteen strokes a minute. Soon, you'll work up to five strokes every ten seconds, or thirty strokes a minute. This is about the speed you want. When this gets too easy, move the tension up a notch. At first, it may slow you down below your thirty stroke per minute pace, but it shouldn't feel too hard. Eventually, you'll get back up to the thirty-stroke pace. When *that* gets too easy, nudge the tension up a bit more. (See Beginner's Indoor Rowing Program on the following page.)

## Intermediate Indoor Rowing

You are an intermediate indoor rower if you can row thirty strokes a minute nonstop for thirty minutes three times a week. If you wish to increase the workout, increase the tension just enough to slow your pace to twenty strokes per minute; then, over a period of weeks, work your way back to thirty strokes per minute. Or stay at the same tension but add five minutes every couple of weeks until you are rowing forty-five minutes nonstop three or four times a week. This should put you into marvelous shape.

## Masters Indoor Rowing

You are a master indoor rower if you row thirty strokes per minute for forty-five minutes nonstop, three or four times a week. To increase the workload, add five minutes every few weeks until you're rowing one hour nonstop. This should turn

## BEGINNER'S INDOOR ROWING PROGRAM

Adjust the tension to the lowest setting. Aim for three strokes every ten seconds, or eighteen strokes per minute.

| WEEK | ROW (IN MINUTES) | REST (IN MINUTES) | REPEATS | TOTAL MINUTES |
|---|---|---|---|---|
| 1 | 1 | 2* | 4 | 12** |
| 2 | 1½ | 2 | 4 | 14 |
| 3 | 1½ | 2 | 4 | 14 |
| 4 | 1½ | 1½ | 5 | 15 |
| 5 | 1½ | 1½ | 6 | 18 |
| 6 | 1½ | 1½ | 6 | 18 |
| 7 | 1½ | 1 | 5 | 15 |
| 8 | 1½ | 1 | 6 | 17½ |
| 9 | 1½ | 1 | 6 | 17½ |
| 10 | 2 | 1½ | 5 | 17½ |
| 11 | 2 | 1½ | 6 | 21 |
| 12 | 2 | 1½ | 6 | 21 |
| 13 | 2 | 1 | 7 | 21 |
| 14 | 2 | 1 | 8 | 24 |
| 15 | 5 | 1 | 4 | 24 |
| 16 | 5 | 1 | 4 | 24 |
| 17 | 10 | 2 | 2 | 24 |
| 18 | 10 | 2 | 2 | 24 |
| 19 | 15 | 2 | 1 | 32 |
| 20 | 30 | 0 | 0 | 30 nonstop |

*Or as long as it takes you to catch your breath.
**Stay at this level until you're comfortable

From now on, row thirty minutes nonstop at lowest tension and eighteen strokes per minute until it feels easy. Then row faster, at twenty or twenty-five strokes per minute, and continue at that pace until it too becomes too easy. Gradually work your way up to thirty strokes per minute for thirty minutes nonstop. When that becomes too easy, tighten the tension just until you can notice the difference, and continue paddling.

you into Super Athlete. If the tension feels too light, crank it tighter—only tight enough, however, to slow you down to twenty-five strokes per minute. This way you won't get so tired that you won't be able to row for the full hour.

# First Aid

We've never heard of anyone hurting themselves on a rower. True, your hands may become blistered if the handles aren't padded with cushiony foam, but this doesn't happen nearly as often with indoor rowing handles as it does on real outdoor oars. If you do get a small blister that doesn't hurt and hasn't popped, gently clean it with soap and water, then leave it alone. Protect it during your workouts with a bandage, piece of moleskin, or a strip of one of the new, breathable, water-filled plastic synthetic skins used to treat burns. Remove the covering and expose the blister to the air as much as possible. If the blister is large, painful, and hasn't popped, clean it thoroughly with soap and water and alcohol or antiseptic. Prick it a few times along the edges with a needle sterilized in a flame. Do not remove the flap of skin—it acts as a painless, sterile dressing. Dry the blister and cover it with a sterile bandage. If the blister has torn or popped, carefully cut away the shredded skin, wash the area, allow it to air-dry, then apply a sterile dressing. If the area becomes reddened or more painful, or if red streaks appear around the blister, see a doctor immediately.

If you don't wear shoes while you row, you'll rub the tops of your feet red and raw against the foot straps.

If you get backaches, either your seat is too high or you're leaning too far back at the end of each stroke.

Indoor rowing, like its outdoor counterpart, is nature's perfect exercise. Row for a half hour three or four times a week, and you'll be firmer, noticeably trimmer, stronger, and much more flexible. You'll also be full of energy, the kind of energy people call vitality, a fluid sort of liveliness. It's hard to imagine anything more rewarding, and when you're done, you don't have to haul your boat out of the water and stow it in your garage. All you have to do is get up and walk into the kitchen for a nice, tall glass of orange juice.

# CHAPTER 9

# Cross-Country Skiing Machines: No Snow, No Chills, No Spills, Great Shape

Cross-country skiing, whether indoors or out, is a study in contradictions. For years, athletes and exercise physiologists have considered cross-country skiing the most perfect aerobic exercise known. Its aerobic potential and its whole-body exercise outstrip even rowing. It strengthens the heart and lungs better than any other sport, trims and firms the whole leg and hips, abdomen, arms, and shoulders. Cross-country skiing (also called Nordic skiing) has one more advantage: because it is such vigorous exercise, you see your progress much sooner than with any other sport. (Cross-country skiing is covered in Chapter 16.)

And yet, as vigorous as it can be, it doesn't have to feel strenuous. You move at your own easy aerobic pace. The fact that you're using so many muscles gives you a superb workout without feeling like you're killing yourself in the process.

For years, cross-country skiers tried to figure out how to ski all year round. Not even people who live in Minnesota get that privilege, and some of the rest of us never see snow. (Some of us who do see snow would rather not exercise in it.) Finally, several years ago, some ingenious inventor came up with an indoor cross-country skiing machine that lets you kick and glide your way to complete physical fitness right in the warmth of your living room. Good skiing machines give you an action very similar to the feeling of skiing on snow: as you stand on the platform, you slide your legs back and forth to imitate the motion of skis on snow, and you pull against cords with your arms to imitate the backward push of ski poles dug into the snow.

# The Pitch

In the last seven years, super-fitness cross-country ski machines have been challenging the sales of the moderate and high-quality cycling and rowing machines, and for two good reasons. First, cross-country skiing is the most productive fitness exercise you can do. Second, cross-country skiing machines simulate all of the effects of Nordic skiing, much better than rowers simulate rowing or exerbikes simulate cycling. These skiing machines tone up *every* major muscle group, give you excellent cardiorespiratory benefits, and do so with no jarring or impact, very little strain, and no stress on your joints. Your posture on a Nordic ski machine is slightly forward, so your back is protected. Therefore, people who have back trouble when they use a rowing machine find skiers quite comfortable. Because you use your arms a little more than your legs, you can spike your heart rate up very high very quickly, which is fine for people in top condition, but not great for people just starting out. However, it is easy to keep the arm exercise down until you're in better shape: either don't use your arms at all, or keep the tension adjustment very low.

**Don't ski indoors without a doctor's approval** if you have severe arthritis in your hands—they may hurt or you simply may not be able to grip the cord handles.

# Buying and Testing Your Equipment

A cross-country skiing exerciser combines two principles: gliding along a track with your feet and pulling against a resistance with your arms. Like any other good quality exerciser, Nordic exercisers are stable, sturdily built, and don't wobble when you glide back and forth or pull hard with your arms.

The exerciser should have foot cups so your foot doesn't slip out while sliding back and forth. Some cheap machines give you just a plate or cushion for your feet. You can't glide as freely this way, because your foot isn't anchored and you can't comfortably lift your heel. Besides, it's dangerous because your foot can—and will—slide off and you can strain an ankle or scrape your skin on the edges of the machine.

The gliding tracks should slide back and forth smoothly and easily without catching somewhere along the line. You should be able to move smoothly from one glide to the next without getting stuck or having to reposition your foot. You should also be able to adjust the resistance along the track so you can ski easily, as if on a flat meadow, or with great effort, as if up Mount McKinley. The adjustment mechanism should be easy to reach, easy to set, and should stay where you put it.

The arm resistance should also be adjustable and should have its own settings separate from the legs. Most good quality skiers use arm cords rather than poles. Arm cords use a flywheel or some other variable resistance mechanism to give you greatest resistance at the beginning of the push and lightest at the end, the way real skiing does. Cheaper machines use poles or levers attached to the bottom platform. Their resistance is uneven, often harder at the middle or end than at the beginning. The arm-cord handles should be padded with something both cushiony and smooth to prevent numbness and blisters.

Good ski machines provide a pelvic cushion to push against as you ski. You don't get the full cross-country skiing workout without it. What's more, it keeps your body aligned and your posture correct; it protects your back; works all your muscles; and trains you for good skiing form, should you want to go from indoor to outdoor skiing someday. No skiing machine without a pelvic cushion is worth the few bucks you'll pay for it.

Beyond that, the choice is up to you and your accountant. Classic ski machines, costing close to $500 at full retail, have clearly marked, easy-to-adjust tension scales, speedometers, and fold up to be stored in a closet. If you want to spend more, you'll find equipment with gadgetry to monitor your heart rate, your tempo, and maybe even your thoughts, for all we know. One bit of advice: Don't buy a machine by mail-order unless you've tried it in a store first.

# Clothing

Wear lightweight, warm-weather clothing. You're going to work up quite a sweat. Shoes are a must or you'll cut or scrape the tops and bottoms of your feet, and you might even catch a toe. However, you don't have to be too particular about the type of shoe, as long as it has a low heel. Since there is no jarring in this activity, you don't need shoes to protect your feet from the assaults common during walking, running, or jumping. Turn on the fan while you're working out—but don't get chilled—and be sure to drink a lot of water before, during, and after you ski.

# Warming Up

Warm up your heart by skiing slowly and easily for five or ten minutes with no resistance on arms or legs. Once you've worked up a sweat, set the resistance for a total workout. If you're stiff the day after a workout, do the No-Stress Super Stretches in Chapter 3 after your aerobic warm-up or during your cool-down. Cool down after skiing by poling and gliding easily at no resistance for another five minutes.

# The Basics

### FIVE-MINUTE LESSON

You'll make faster progress on a skiing machine than you do on many other exercisers, because you can adjust the tension on the skis and the ski poles separately; because you can ski very slowly and still get a workout; and because the movements are so smooth.

In order to understand how to use a skiing machine, you must understand how real cross-country skiing feels. When you ski in snow, you reach forward with, say, your right ski pole, dig it into the snow, and then pull yourself forward with it while you push down and back with your left ski. (Your right ski and left pole come forward at the same time, but they're not doing any work.) When you're done pushing with your right pole, your left arm takes over, planting its pole and pulling you forward as you push backward with your right leg. Your legs do all their work on the backward slide; sliding forward again is just gravy. The same goes for your arms: they do all their work on the backward push and none as they come forward again.

First, adjust the tension on the skis and the ski poles. Experiment. Leave it at zero, where it was set during your warm-up, and see if you start to huff and puff. If not, turn up the tension on the legs a bit. For the time being, though, leave the ski pole tension at zero, because arms are weaker than legs. (In addition, doing too much arm work spikes up your heart rate too high too soon.) Move the pelvic pad up or down so that it contacts your pelvis at hip joint level.

Start out machine-skiing without the poles. Fit your feet into the ski straps. The straps hold the ball of your foot steady but allow you to move your heel up and down freely. Hold onto the handlebars for balance and lean with much of your weight against the hip pad. Put all your weight on your right ski. Push against the hip pad so that your right ski pushes backward. As the right ski reaches the rear extent of its range, lift your heel up, let the weight come off it (but don't actually lift the foot off the ski), and transfer your weight to your left ski. Slide your right ski forward again with your toe as you push against the hip pad and slide the left ski back. The balls of your feet never lift off the skis.

The hip pad push is crucial. You're not actually sliding your foot backward. You're just keeping your weight on that foot while you push against the pad. When you push against the pad, your body pushes the ski backward. If you feel as if you're jogging, you're skiing wrong. Lean against the hip pad more.

Keep skiing without poling until it feels comfortable. This may take a few minutes or a few days. It probably won't take weeks the way it does with other sports, but if it does, who cares? Every moment you're practicing, you're getting a superb aerobic workout, and eventually, you'll find it delightfully easy.

Now add the arms. (Remember to turn the tension all the way down. Keep the work your arms and legs do at a comfortable huffing-and-puffing point.) Grasp the ski pole grips and reach far forward with, say, your right arm as you slide your right ski backward. Pull your ski pole back until your hand is far behind your body. The first part of the pull will take most of the effort; the second half of the backward swing and all of the forward arc is a breeze. Keep your arms and legs in opposition: when you're poling back with your right arm, your left ski is sliding back and your right ski is coming forward. As you reach the rearmost swing of your arm, swing your left hand forward so you can start pulling back with your left hand and sliding forward on your left foot. Keep your elbows slightly bent.

## SCHEDULE

Once you coordinate arms and legs, ski slowly, going about three to four miles per hour on the machine's speedometer. (That's about five to six kilometers per hour on machines with metric speedometers.) The first week, you may be able to ski for a maximum of eight minutes nonstop at a time. That's fine. Do that four times the first week. The second week, try to ski two nonstop eight-minute intervals, resting for a couple of minutes in between, either by sliding without poling or stopping altogether. As you start to progress, add a few minutes each week (or each day if you're improving quickly), and try to keep the rest periods down to one minute, if possible.

Aim at skiing at least twenty minutes and a maximum of thirty minutes nonstop, three or four times a week. As your condition becomes better still, speed up.

The first week or two, ski without using your arms, until you're comfortable; then add your arms. When you can ski using both arms and legs, begin the following program, skiing no more than three or four miles per hour. Ski three or four times a week. Rest by sliding without poling or stopping altogether.

## BEGINNER'S INDOOR CROSS-COUNTRY
## SKIING PROGRAM

| WEEK | SKI (IN MINUTES) | REST (IN MINUTES) | REPEATS | TOTAL SKIING TIME IN MINUTES |
|------|------------------|-------------------|---------|------------------------------|
| 1 | 8 | | 1 | 8 |
| 2 | 8 | 2 | 2 | 16 |
| 3 | 8 | 1 | 2 | 16 |
| 4 | 10 | 1 | 2 | 20 |
| 5 | 12 | 1 | 2 | 24 |
| 6 | 15 | 2 | 1 | 20 |
| | 5 | | | |
| 7 | 15 | 1 | 1 | 20 |
| | 5 | | | |
| 8 | 18 | 2 | 1 | 24 |
| | 6 | | | |
| 9 | 18 | 1 | 1 | 24 |
| | 6 | | | |
| 10 | 20 | | | 20 |

If this schedule moves too quickly for you, repeat the even-numbered weeks as many times as necessary.

If this schedule moves too slowly for you, eliminate weeks 3, 5, 7, and 9.

Once you can ski for twenty minutes nonstop, stay at this level until it no longer makes you huff and puff. Then gradually increase the speed until you're skiing about eight miles per hour. When that feels too easy, increase the tension first on the skiis and then on the poles.

---

# Intermediate Indoor Skiing

You are an intermediate indoor skier if you can ski thirty minutes nonstop three or four times a week. As your condition becomes better still, speed up. Remember, you should always work at a huffing-and-puffing pace. You get more of an aerobic workout by speeding up your pace than by tightening the tension adjustments. An eight-mile-per-hour (or thirteen-kilo-meters-per-hour) speed is ideal. When this seems too easy, don't speed up any more. Instead, tighten the resistance—first on the skis and then on the poles.

When this becomes too easy, add five minutes of skiing every couple of weeks until you're skiing forty-five minutes nonstop.

## Masters Indoor Skiing

You are a master indoor skier if you can ski at an eight-mile-per-hour pace for forty-five minutes nonstop, three or four times a week. To increase your workload, add five minutes every few weeks to work yourself up to one hour of nonstop skiing. After that, whenever your workout feels too easy, inten-sify the resistance, first on your skis and then on your poles.

## First Aid

This is a trouble-free sport. Blisters on your hands are about the only injury you're likely to get, and even they are rare. See the First Aid section in Chapter 8, for home treatment of blisters.

There's something poetically enthralling about a cross-country skiing machine. The design is ingenious—it just feels good to stand on the thing. The exercise is only as demanding as you want it to be, and yet it makes you as healthy and happy as any aerobic exercise can. And the results are a miracle to behold in your mirror—just about every muscle in your body trim, slim, and supple. These machines may not be cheap, but they are well worth the investment.

# CHAPTER 10

# Treadmills for Walking and Running: Take a Hike Without Leaving Home

**W**alk or run on a treadmill in your rumpus room and you'll get all the benefits of walking or running outdoors except the smell of the flowers on a warm summer's day. (So buy yourself a bouquet of roses, and you'll have it all.) Walking, as you'll discover in Chapter 12, gives you a wonderfully unstressful aerobic workout, leaving you with all the blessings of aerobics—weight loss, cardiorespiratory health, mood-lifting, and the rest—without a lot of effort. Running, if you're built for it, works faster and is almost as aerobic.

You might expect to lose something when you translate four-mile walks through the city streets into forty-five-minute hikes on a conveyor belt, but don't worry. You don't lose a thing, because walking and running involve such simple, uncomplicated movements. Walking or running on a treadmill gives you the same benefits as walking or running through the streets of your neighborhood. In fact, the scale tips a little in favor of the treadmill.

When you walk or run outside, you get some health-giving fresh air—assuming it's not too polluted. But that's just about everything in favor of outdoor leg work. The sidewalk is hard

116

and causes jarring injuries. Your route may be too full of hills for a beginning runner or may have none of the hills an advanced walker needs. The treadmill, in contrast, is cushioned, so it reduces the jarring, pounding impact on your legs and spine. It lets you choose when you want to run up or down a hill (all you do is turn a dial). But then again, the outdoors is free to all. Treadmills are quite expensive. Score: two to two, but tilting toward treadmills.

We're not going to devote as much space to treadmills as to other exercise machines. First of all, they are too expensive for most people. Prices start about $500 for nonmotorized treadmills—and you don't get much for that investment—then shoot up to around $2,000 and up (mostly up) for moderate and good-quality motorized versions. Second, neither running nor walking are full-body exercises. They give you a good aerobic workout, but not such a good workout that they're worth the expense. Third and finally, treadmills are bulky and almost impossible to hide. If you buy a treadmill, figure on giving up a room.

**A note on rebounders and mini-tramps.** These devices are called by many names. The most descriptive is mini-trampolines, but they're also sold as rebounders, jogging tramps, and bouncers. Whatever you call them, they're a lot of fun but don't do much for your physical condition. If you're in poor shape, bouncing or jogging on a mini-tramp will get you huffing and puffing enough for a fair workout. But as soon as your condition improves—say, after a month or so of bouncing three or four times a week—you get many fewer aerobic and toning benefits than from plain walking. (For example, a group of women in one study jogged on a rebounder for thirty minutes a day, five days a week, for twelve weeks. Their aerobic fitness improved a paltry 4.5 percent. They lost no body fat, and their serum cholesterol and endurance levels stayed at their pre-exercise levels.)

# The Pitch

Walking is a purely aerobic exercise—perhaps the purest. It builds your heart and lungs and strengthens your legs. Running is also aerobic exercise, but you also do some nonaerobic exercise during every step. It too strengthens your legs. Neither one does anything for your upper body. Walking and running on a treadmill give you the same benefits as walking and running outdoors.

**Don't walk on a treadmill without a doctor's approval if** you have Ménière's disease or any other type of dizziness or balance problem.

**Don't run on a treadmill without a doctor's approval if** you have heart disease, high blood pressure, or high cholesterol levels, or if you have knee, neck, or lower back problems, arthritis, or osteoporosis.

## Buying and Testing Your Equipment

Treadmills come in two varieties: nonmotorized and motorized. On a nonmotorized treadmill, your steps turn a large, wide belt, much the way a laboratory rat's little steps turn the treadmill in its cage. A motorized treadmill moves for you, but that doesn't make it any easier because you've still got to walk or run at the speed of the treadmill or you'll fall down.

Any treadmill should be sturdily built, stable, and unwobbly. The belt should move smoothly with no jerking or catching. The surface should be well cushioned, the tread should be substantial so that it will hold up to constant use, and it should have sturdy handles or side rails to grab if you stumble.

Motorized treadmills should have easy-to-set adjustments so you can change the speed and grade. When you stiffen the resistance on the grade adjustment, you feel like you're walking uphill. They should also have emergency cutoff switches within easy reach from anywhere on the treadmill.

To increase the speed of a nonmotorized treadmill, walk or run faster. To create a makeshift grade on nonmotorized treadmills, place boards under the front end to tilt it up. Although this isn't the safest arrangement—if you're not careful, the treadmill will fall off the boards with disastrous results —it does have one advantage. Clinging onto the handles of a tilted nonmotorized treadmill builds up some upper-body strength. However, because you're pushing a belt as well as striding along, nonmotorized treadmills tend to irritate your feet.

# Clothing

Wear lightweight clothes and shoes and aim a fan in your direction if you get hot. Drink plenty of water before, during, and after your walk or run.

# Warming Up

Warm up your heart and lungs by walking slowly at zero grade for five or ten minutes until you're huffing and puffing. If you run, you may need a warm-up stretch after your aerobic warm-up. (See discussion in Chapter 3.) Get off the treadmill and do the No-Stress Super Stretches in Chapter 3. Cool down your heart with another five- or ten-minute walk on flat terrain. If you feel achy after your cool-down, do the No-Stress Super Stretches again.

# The Basics

Follow the walking or running programs in Part Three. Start out slowly (at a pace of perhaps two and a half or three miles per hour) with no resistance, and increase your speed every time the workout becomes too easy. Increase the grade when you are walking faster than four miles an hour or running faster than seven miles an hour.

# First Aid

You're subject to the same aches and pains on a treadmill as you are on city streets: blisters on your feet; aches down the backs of your legs or in your shins or groin; sharp pains, cramps, or numbness in your calves; pain in your knees; shoulder or side stitches. See the First Aid section in Chapter 12.

Sure, treadmills are expensive and gobble up space. And sure, you can get the same benefits by walking or running outdoors. Still, many of us love to work out on a treadmill parked in front of the television. It doesn't feel like we're exercising at all. The machine hums along, our bodies hum along, and all of a sudden our thirty or sixty minutes are up and we didn't even notice them passing. Overall, we don't consider that a bad bargain.

# C H A P T E R   1 1

# Jump Ropes: An Exercise You Won't Want to Skip

We've saved the cheapest, most playful—and most strenuous—indoor exercise for last.

Rope skipping will never become an Olympic event. No one—except perhaps the double Dutch championship teams in New York—would even call it a sport. And yet it is one of the most addictive exercises there is. When you skip for a half hour or hour nonstop, you go into a kind of meditative trance. When you come out of your trance, you can add arm cross-overs, high jumps, twirls, and red-hot-peppers for variety, just like the boxers do.

It's easy to learn to jump rope. Every woman probably remembers how from her schoolyard days, and most men can get the hang of it after a few tries.

Skipping rope (step-hopping) is very demanding—too demanding, in fact, if you're not already in pretty good shape. (Jumping over the rope with both feet at the same time, by the way, is even more strenuous. We don't recommend it.) If you skip longer than fifteen minutes nonstop, it builds good aerobic stamina. However, you're going to have to invest several weeks of practice before you can skip long enough to get any aerobic payoff. Although most other sports give you much quicker results, the soothing, intensely meditative quality of skipping rope makes all the effort worthwhile.

You may have heard that skipping rope for ten minutes equals thirty minutes of jogging. Alas, it's not true. Skipping rope for ten minutes is indeed more tiring than jogging for ten minutes, but that's because you're building up the lactic acid wastes we described in Chapter 3. After the nonaerobic phase, skipping rope nets about the same aerobic benefits as running, minute for minute.

# The Pitch

Skipping rope is great aerobic exercise *once you get past the first ten or fifteen minutes.* It improves the strength and endurance of your legs but does little for your upper arms unless you use a weighted or long-handled jump rope. At first glance, skipping rope may appear to violate the aerobic rule that you must cover ground, but that's only true at the beginning level. After that, you can skip along a homemade path, and then your large leg muscles pull you across a space as much as they do in any of the other sports in Parts Two and Three. If you have a large enough room in your house, try skipping in a wide circle or oval. If you don't have the room, try skipping around the high-school running track or down a quiet side street.

Skipping rope may be too strenuous for some. It spikes up your heart rate very quickly, as any fast arm exercise does, and it's impossible to start skipping and turning the rope slowly since a slow rope won't go over your head; it just collapses in a heap at your feet.

Good jump ropes cost peanuts compared to just about any other sports equipment. And they don't take up extra room.

**Don't skip rope without a doctor's approval** if you have any heart or circulatory problems, or if you have arthritis in your knees, hips, or back.

# Equipment

Jump ropes cost anywhere from three dollars for a superior homemade model to thirty-five dollars for weighted and long-handled versions. Any jump rope should be thick (5/16 to 3/8 inch in diameter) and heavy enough to go over your head in a smooth arc. It should be long enough for your height. To measure, stand on the center of the rope and pull each side up toward your shoulders. The rope, not counting the handles, should come a bit past your armpits. The rope should hit the floor on each swing while your body is straight and your hands are at hip level. Too short is impossible, but too long is fixable. Just tie a few knots in the rope. (With knots, be extra careful when you jump; getting hit by a knot is like getting hit by a rock from a slingshot.)

The handles of any jump rope should turn smoothly and effortlessly. Stiff ropes give you sore wrists. Some handles have ball bearings to keep them moving smoothly. Make sure the handle itself feels silky as a baby's bottom or you'll end up with blisters. Some fancy ropes come with extra-long handles. They are supposed to strengthen your arms while you jump. You can get the same effect by using your whole arm to swing the rope in wide circles. (Usually, you turn just with your wrists.) Some handles have built-in counters to record the number of revolutions you've made. Each revolution equals a jump.

We prefer our homemade rope to almost every commercial product. You cut it to the length you and you alone need (an important factor for very short or very tall people) and then install grips that fit your hand perfectly. Start with thick but pliable rope. Sash cord, old-fashioned cotton clothesline, or hemp rope from the local hardware store will do, but we prefer ¾-inch-diameter nylon line from a marine supply shop. Buy at least a foot more than you think you'll need. Test the length by standing on it, as we mentioned above, or buy a length double your height—twelve feet for a six-foot person, for example.

For handles, you want some sort of durable tube: four- or five-inch sections of aluminum or plastic pipe, cannoli tubes (molds for an Italian fried pastry), or (our favorite) sections of rigid Lucite tubing. The tube should be wide enough to allow the rope to turn freely inside it, and it should be firm enough that you won't crush it when you grip it. Thread two tubes onto the rope, one at each end, tie knots in each end, and start skipping. You don't have to tie a knot on the other side of the handles because the swinging rope holds them in place.

Your floor is almost as important a piece of equipment as

your rope. Skip on something with some spring to it. A bare old-fashioned hardwood floor laid over subflooring and joists (rather than concrete) is ideal. You get enough bounce to cushion your feet and absorb some of the skipping shock to your legs. A wall-to-wall carpet is second-best. It does a good job of cushioning, but its uneven surface may cause you to twist your ankle. Do not skip on loose rugs: you're sure to trip and fall. Do not skip on concrete floors: they offer no cushioning and are likely to give you shin splints, knee pain, bruised feet, and many other injuries.

# Clothing

Wear very lightweight clothing and good aerobic or running shoes. The shoes will cushion the balls of your feet and keep you from catching your feet in the rope. Women should wear good supportive bras. Cool yourself with a fan—you're going to work up quite a sweat—and drink plenty of water before, during, and after skipping.

# Warming Up

The biggest disadvantage to skipping rope is that you can't warm up for it by skipping slowly. The slowest you can jump is about seventy-six turns a minute, and that's already too fast for a warm-up. Warm up your heart and lungs by walking, bouncing, or dancing around the house for five minutes or by skipping (with the rope) as slowly as possible for half a minute, resting for half a minute, skipping for half a minute, and so on. (At first, you won't be able to skip for more than thirty seconds anyway, so this will come naturally.)

Skipping rope is one of the few exercises that demand warm-up stretches. Whether you also have to do the No-Stress Super Stretches (see Chapter 3) after your aerobic workout depends on whether you got sore the last time you skipped. To cool down, repeat whatever you did to warm up. If you're stiff or if you get sore the next day, do the No-Stress Super Stretches again. Whatever you do, be sure to cool your heart down by walking or prancing about the house for five or ten minutes after each skipping session.

# The Basics

## FIVE-MINUTE LESSON

If you've never skipped rope before, skip without a rope first. Step, then do a little hop on one foot, then step and do a little hop on the other. That's skipping. Get yourself to the point where you can skip without falling over your own feet, stopping whenever necessary to catch your breath, but otherwise aiming for a rate of seventy-five to eighty skips per minute. Bounce gently on the balls of your feet and push off with your toes. Don't land flat-footed. Keep your knees very slightly bent and lift them only a half-inch or so off the floor.

When you feel relaxed and fluid as you skip, add the rope but don't jump over it yet. Hold both handles in one hand and turn the rope at your side while you skip. Try to turn as many times as you skip. Keep your elbows tucked in close to your body and use your wrist, not your whole arm, to turn the rope.

When this feels comfortable, put it all together. With a handle in each hand, turn the rope at the same pace as you skip. Be economical with your movements: turn with your wrists, bounce on your toes. Swing the rope, step-hop over it; swing the rope, step-hop over it (see Figure 11.1). Hop just high enough to clear the rope.

Each foot should land in the same spot time after time. If this skipping rhythm is too hard for you to coordinate at first, jump over the rope once, jogging instead of skipping. Do this only as a last resort, however, because it's twice as strenuous and twice as jarring as skipping is.

Keep your body erect, and look straight ahead of you, not at your feet. Turn the rope as slowly as you can and still keep it moving.

## SCHEDULE

Start as slowly as possible, and jump until you feel very winded. Then stop and walk around to catch your breath a bit, skip some more, catch your breath, and so on for a few minutes. The first few weeks, you'll probably be able to jump only for thirty seconds or a minute. That's fine. You'll build up endurance very quickly, and the first time you jump a full minute,

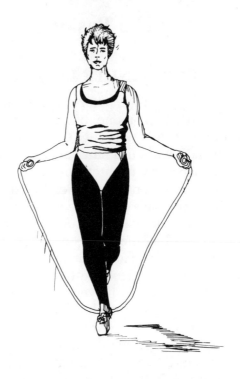

FIGURE 11.1  ROPE SKIPPING.

you'll be so proud, you'll want to rush out and announce it to the neighborhood.

After the first few weeks, as you've built up a bit of stamina, follow this pattern. Try to increase the length of time you skip rope before you run out of steam, and try to decrease the amount of time it takes you to recover between jumping bouts. Every two weeks, add another minute to your total jumping time. During the first of those two weeks, allow yourself two minutes to rest between each interval. During the second of those two weeks, allow yourself to rest for only one minute between intervals.

After a while, you'll be able to jump nonstop for five minutes, then six, then seven . . . and you'll feel an enormous sense of accomplishment. Work yourself up to two fifteen-minute intervals, first with a two-minute rest period in between, then with a one-minute rest. Your goal is to jump a total of thirty minutes nonstop three times a week. This is all you need for a basic aerobic workout.

## BEGINNER'S ROPE-SKIPPING PROGRAM

| WEEK | SKIP (IN MINUTES) | REST (IN MINUTES) | REPEATS | TOTAL SKIPPING TIME IN MINUTES |
|---|---|---|---|---|
| 1 | ½ | 2 | 6 | 3* |
| 2 | ½ | 2 | 6 | 3 |
| 3 | 1 | 2 | 3 | 3 |
| 4 | 1 | 1 | 3 | 3 |
| 5 | 1 | 2 | 4 | 4 |
| 6 | 1 | 1 | 4 | 4 |
| 7 | 1½ 2 | 2 | 2 | 5 |
| 8 | 1½ 2 | 1 | 2 | 5 |
| 9 | 2 | 2 | 3 | 6 |
| 10 | 2 | 1 | 3 | 6 |
| 11 | 2 3 | 2 | 2 | 7 |
| 12 | 2 3 | 1 | 2 | 7 |
| 13 | 3 2 | 2 | 2 | 8 |
| 14 | 3 2 | 1 | 2 | 8 |
| 15 | 3 | 2 | 3 | 9 |
| 16 | 4 | 1 | 3 | 12** |
| 17 | 5 | 1 | 3 | 15 |
| 18 | 6 | 1 | 3 | 18 |
| 19 | 7 | 1 | 3 | 21 |
| 20 | 8 | 1 | 3 | 24 |

*Stay at this—and any—level until you are comfortable.
**The pace picks up here. If this is too fast, allow yourself two minutes between intervals and stay at each level for two weeks.

From now on, add a minute to each interval every week. Do three skipping intervals, with one-minute rest periods between, so that your total time increases by three minutes each

**Beginner's Rope-Skipping Program,** continued

week. When you reach three ten-minute skipping intervals, for a total of thirty minutes, stay there for a couple of weeks to become adjusted to this pace. Then, keep your total skipping minutes at thirty, but work yourself up to two fifteen-minute intervals (nonstop) with one- or two-minute rest stops in between. When you get to the point where you can skip for fifteen minutes nonstop, rest for one minute then skip another fifteen minutes nonstop, and stay at this level for another few weeks. The cut out the rest interval completely and skip thirty minutes nonstop.

If this schedule moves too quickly, spend two or three weeks—or as many as you need to be comfortable—at each level. If it moves too slowly, cut out the week with the two-minute rest periods.

---

# Intermediate Rope Skipping

You are an intermediate rope skipper when you already have been skipping for thirty minutes nonstop, three times a week, for several months. If your session becomes too easy or if you would enjoy skipping longer, add ten minutes every two or three weeks until you're up to forty-five minutes.

Skipping rope this way in your living room or rumpus room is very effective aerobic exercise, but if you want it to approach aerobic perfection, cover ground as you skip.

You have a few options. The easiest, least demanding, and most convenient solution is to move in an oval—a sort of miniature running track—as you skip. Even a course of eight or ten feet each direction is fine. If you can't manage this without bumping into furniture or wearing out the rug, perhaps your garage or backyard will work. If not, try skipping along a quiet side street. The street is better than the sidewalk because it is usually softer and smoother and because your rope is less likely to get caught in overhanging trees. Beware of cars.

Covering distance while skipping rope is hard work. At first, skip forward a few feet, then skip in place until you feel rested, then skip forward a few feet, and so on. Every week, skip farther and rest less. Within a few weeks, you'll be skipping forward the entire session.

# Masters Rope Skipping

You are a master rope skipper when you can skip for forty-five minutes nonstop, moving across a distance the whole time.

# First Aid

**Pain in the ankles or shins during or after skipping:** You may be working on too soft a surface or wearing shoes that are too soft.

**Bruised feeling on bottoms of feet:** You're jumping on a surface that's too hard.

**Blisters:** Most blisters are caused when your foot rubs up and down inside your sock or shoe. Some may come from skipping on hard surfaces. See the First Aid section in Chapter 8.

**Shin splints:** Hot, searing pain and tenderness anywhere along your shinbone from ankle to knee; pain eases an hour or so after you stop skipping. The term *shin splints* refers to injuries to several parts of the bone, tendons, or muscle casing. You've been skipping on hard surfaces longer than your legs can tolerate and they're sending you messages to do something . . . quick.

Apply ice packs for ten minutes every few hours for the first two days. Compression (by means of an elastic bandage) sometimes helps, as does elevation. Stretch your calf muscles and your Achilles tendon (just above the heel) but don't stretch your shins; that will only make your shin splints worse. If they're mild, they may go away after a few more minutes of jumping. If they're very painful, give up skipping rope for a while and try a non–weight-bearing sport such as exercise bicycling, rowing, or swimming. After a couple of weeks, try skipping again.

If the shin splints recur, try one or more of the following: Stretch your calves before each session. Wear heel lifts. Wear cushioned inner soles. Find a hardwood or carpeted floor to jump on. Wear high socks to keep your muscles warm. Find another sport. If the outside of your calf swells up or hardens or if the pain lasts longer than two hours after an exercise session, see a doctor.

**Knee pain:** Apply ice packs for ten minutes every few hours for a couple of days. Elevate the knee or wear an elastic bandage for those first two days, but don't wear the bandage too long or you'll weaken the muscles around your knee and cause further injury. Do hamstring and calf stretches. Stretch the bottoms of your feet by rolling your feet over a beer can or soda bottle for five minutes or so, three times a day. Try wearing arch supports or heel wedges in your shoes.

**Stabbing, searing, or dull pain in side or shoulder:** A stitch or catch in the side. There are several causes: a spasm of the diaphragm muscle caused by heavy breathing and inadequate supply of oxygen; spasm of one of the abdominal muscles, again from insufficient oxygen; intestinal gas; unusually intense contractions of the intestinal wall. Stitches also occur in the neck or middle or lower chest and are often difficult for the layperson to distinguish from a heart attack. If home treatment doesn't work or if you're worried you're having a heart attack, see your doctor.

Try one or more of the following: Bend over at the waist, raise your knee on the side that hurts, and press the stitch with your fingers. Or lie on your back and raise your arms above your head. Or hold your nose, purse your lips and blow out, resisting the stream of air with your lips. Or find a position in which you can grab the knee on the side that hurts and pull it toward your chest with one hand while pressing the stitch with the fingers of your other hand. To prevent recurrence, make a pit stop before you exercise. Don't eat gassy foods. Stretch your abdominal muscles after your aerobic warm-up.

Breathe the way nature intended—inflating your abdomen instead of your chest. Most people breathe backward—when they take a deep breath, their chests swell while their bellies stay fairly still. Take this test: Stand up and put one hand on your chest and one on your abdomen. Take a deep breath. If the hand on your chest moves more than the hand on your abdomen, your diaphragm is going up instead of down on each breath and you're breathing backward. It'll take you a few days to unlearn this bad habit, but once you get the hang of proper breathing, it will become natural. Practice by lying down on your back and placing a heavy book on your abdomen. Put one hand on your chest. Each time you take a deep breath, make sure the book moves up and the hand on your chest doesn't. By the way, you get a welcome bonus here. Not only will this exercise train you to take genuinely deep breaths, perhaps for the first time in your life, but it will also strengthen and tighten your abdominal muscles.

Skipping rope, like running, isn't for everyone, but if you enjoy it and if it feels good, you'll discover, as we have, the delicious rapture of hopping over that rope, 4,500 times an hour, without ever missing a step. Our problems melt away. Solutions to worries just pop into our heads. And, at the end of our workout, we actually enjoy returning to the real world of work and family.

And we'll tell you this: there's nothing like the thrill of passing some kids jumping rope on the street and jumping in and going several rounds of Teddy Bear, Teddy Bear with them. If that doesn't make you feel young, nothing will.

# PART

# THREE

## Exercising Outdoors

**O**utdoors, you're not just exercising to exercise. You're walking or swimming or skiing as much for the joy as for the health of it. You feel the sun on your skin, you smell the wind, you hear the buzzing of life on a spring day.

This section of *Going the Distance* explores the eight most aerobic, most beneficial, easiest to learn outdoor sports. We're partisans of them all. When we're swimming, we pity the sweaty walkers making their way down summery city streets. When we're walking, we're sorry for the poor swimmers who can't smell the roses or feel the wind in their hair. When we're kayaking, we don't understand why anyone would want to struggle with two oars instead of one light paddle, and when we're rowing, we can't fathom why anyone would paddle an inefficient glorified canoe. When we're cycling, we really feel for the poor souls bound by their two feet when they could be exploring miles and miles of countryside in the same amount of time. And when we're skiing, we can't imagine anything more glorious.

It's all a matter of taste. You may love one sport and hate

the next. Read through these chapters until something catches your eye. Then try it. Or try everything. Once you find something you like, stick with it—it'll only get better as the months and years go on.

This is as good a place as any to face one ticklish fact. We would be less than candid if we didn't admit that every one of us, at one time or another, has a bad day. Or ten. Count on it: it'll happen to you. Someday you're going to wake up and not want to exercise.

Don't be too hard on yourself. If you tell yourself that missing a day is a sign of failure and proof of what a rotten person you are, you're going to hate your sport and yourself and give up for good. Everyone has down periods. Even though we know how good a brisk walk will feel, sometimes we still can't get ourselves off the couch and out the door. It's natural to resist anything that takes effort. Nature programmed us that way. We instinctively try to conserve energy, as if we were prehistoric human beings who didn't know where our next meal was coming from.

If you stop blaming yourself and see these obstacles as just a couple of hurdles you have to jump, you can come up with solutions. First ask yourself whether you really like the sport you chose. Does it make you feel good, and are you comfortable doing it? People choose activities for a variety of reasons. You might choose to bicycle because you loved it as a kid and doing it again makes you feel young. You might choose to swim because you never learned how as a kid and it's something you've always dreamed of. You might choose to run because you want to run with a spouse or a friend who's already an accomplished runner. You might choose to row on a machine indoors because you want to exercise in privacy.

When your choice is right, you know it. You glow with the enormous satisfaction of knowing you're accomplishing something. But you may not choose correctly the first time around. You may discover, after all, that you hate to swim. Or that it's not fun to bicycle on busy city streets. Or that running hurts your knees and you only did it to please your wife anyway. The answer is simple: Try another sport. There's something here you're going to love, and you'll learn the second sport more quickly than the first because you're in better shape now.

If you like what you're doing but it's getting a little flat, remind yourself *why* you wanted to exercise in the first place. Get out a piece of paper and write down your goals. Then, write down the progress you've made. We suggest you keep a kind of log so you can see your improvement month after month, year after year. How far could you walk last month? How far—and how fast—are you walking this month? How much did you weigh three months ago? How much do you weigh now? Remember how winded you were climbing the stairs to your friends' hillside home? Do you get winded now? It's easy to lose sight of these gradual, daily changes, but reviewing your fitness record every month or so reminds you how far you've come and makes you want to continue.

It's also natural to resist the intrusions exercise makes on your routine. You're busy. You have work, family, household duties, hobbies, friends, chores, errands, vacations, movies to see. . . . How do you fit exercise into your schedule?

Even if you work at home, fitting in exercise may be complicated, but it's possible. Swim during your lunch break. Walk after dinner. Ride your bike to and from work. Use your cross-country skiing machine while watching the evening news. Get up an hour earlier and row first thing in the morning.

In fact, choosing the time you exercise is one of the most important decisions you'll make. Some people simply can't exercise in the morning—it takes them three cups of coffee just to be able to bend over and put on their socks. Others run out of steam by 4:00 P.M. and could no more swim laps in late afternoon than dance all night. Know thyself and go with the flow.

Invite your spouse to exercise with you. Those thirty or sixty minutes, away from telephones and other distractions and intrusions, may become the time when you talk out your plans and problems. Or exercise with a friend. When you exercise with someone else, each of you urges the other on to keep going when interest flags. And the conversation makes the hour go much more quickly.

Consider organizing your own five- or six-person walking or cycling or whatever club. Members take turns as weekly director, responsible for choosing interesting routes and providing refreshments.

Some people find doing the same thing every day— cycling the same route or swimming in the same pool—is most comforting. They know how far they've gone and exactly what to expect. They enjoy observing the small changes in familiar scenery. All this makes the time go faster. Others need variety—walking tours of new neighborhoods, canoeing along unknown bits of bayshore. Again, know thyself: figure out what you like and do it.

People develop all sorts of tactics to stay involved. One woman we know takes lessons to improve her skills or to learn a new stroke when swimming laps gets a little old. Another woman speedwalks every Sunday with a local club in addition to her daily four-mile walks. A couple we know set off on a cycling tour of France when cycling around town went a bit flat. Another friend went out for a masters rowing team and competes in age-graded regattas throughout his state.

One other ploy is to do more than one kind of exercise. Walk, say, on Monday, Wednesday, and Friday, and take a bicycle ride along a country road on Saturday afternoon. Or swim on weekends and ride an exercise bicycle at the company gym on two or three weekdays. You know how stimulating variety is. What you may not know is that it's wonderful for your body. Doing more than one sport balances your body; the second sport strengthens the muscles the first sport overlooks.

An active life is a joyous circle. You find something you like to do, and the more you do it, the better you feel, and the better you feel, the more you like to do it. Experiment. Eventually you'll settle down to one, two, or three favorites, and you'll discover the exhilaration of moving. It's the best present you can give yourself.

# C H A P T E R  1 2

# Walking: All Things to All People

$\mathcal{S}$urely this has happened to you. You're sitting with your in-laws on Thanksgiving and are about to jump out of your skin. You have an overwhelming urge to take a walk. You get antsier and antsier. So, what the heck, you walk out the door and just down the street. Sure feels good to be out in the fresh air. You keep going, just another block or two, then another and another. After about fifteen minutes, you feel better, and when you come back, forty-five minutes later, you're a new person—mellow, relaxed, cheerful. Nothing bothers you.

You've just bathed in the glow of aerobics, and all you did was take a walk. Yet tell people that walking is the best aerobic exercise they can do, and they shake their heads in disbelief. "Can't be," they protest. "Walking simply isn't hard enough work to be good exercise. It defies the Puritan work ethic."

We're so used to thinking of running as the only aerobic exercise that walking seems too good to be true. Nonetheless, walking wins hands down if you're looking for pure aerobics. If you step out briskly and purposefully, you get *all* the aerobic benefits of, say, running, with none of the unpleasant side effects.

# The Pitch

Let's look in detail at the benefits of walking.

- You burn the same number of calories walking a mile as running a mile (about 100 calories for a 150-pound man; less for a 150-pound woman). It just takes longer to do it.
- Walking is nonjarring. Because one foot is always on the ground when you walk, you don't fall victim to those scary statistics about how three to five times your body weight comes down on your foot with every running step. A little more than half of your body weight comes down on your foot with each walking step, the way nature intended, so you can forget shin splints, muscle cramps, and back problems.
- Walking tones up both the upper *and* lower body muscles as long as you pump forcefully. Ordinary running develops only the back leg muscles.
- You get a good workout from walking no matter what condition you're in.
- Because you are unlikely to hurt yourself walking, you're likely to stick with it. You don't need expensive lessons, special equipment, or perfect weather. With sensible clothing, in fact, you can walk all year around, except during hurricanes or tornadoes.

Walking can perform miracles. Ellen Klein, an "ageless" Spanish translator (we'd guess she's in her mid-fifties), was about fifty pounds overweight. "Like everyone else, I dieted, I fasted on that liquid protein stuff—and my hair fell out," she recalls. "I lost weight on every diet. I gained it back every time. Finally, I got diabetes and my doctor got worried. She referred me to a research project on whether exercise really helps you lose weight better than dieting.

"They broke us up into three groups. My group walked for half an hour a day. There was a group that walked for an hour and a group that didn't walk at all. Our group had to show up at the university every day and go for a walk with one of the researchers. We weren't put on a diet. They just told us not to pig out. I figured that if I didn't pig out, I might lose a little weight, but it would come off so slowly, I'd be ninety before I got thin.

"I lost about a pound a week. Sometimes two or three, but not often. The women in the no-walking group didn't lose much of anything, but the women in the one-hour walking group lost two or three pounds a week. I was so jealous.

"I lost fifty pounds in less than a year, and I've kept on walking and I've kept the weight off."

Walking's not just for the very out of shape. Jerome Trump, a fifty-two-year-old chef in a large Houston restaurant, ran almost every afternoon for six years. "I started running to keep my weight down, but I never really liked it. Still, it worked, so I kept at it. But then I got shin splints. And then a heel spur. And then a stress fracture. And my knees started hurting for the first time since high school.

"Then, about a year ago, I started seeing all this stuff about walking in the papers and magazines. I ignored it, because I figured walking couldn't do nearly as much as running, but then I noticed more and more people walking, not running. And they weren't just old guys. They were people my age and a whole lot younger. I was getting to the point where I dreaded tying on my shoes each day, so I thought I'd give it a try. The first day, I just walked pretty fast, and I barely broke a sweat. The next day, I strapped on some wrist weights and had a good time. I've been walking ever since."

Walking is all things to all people: a leisurely stroll around the block, or an Olympic sport—racewalking—full of seven-minute miles; a long contemplative walk, or an intense workout with weights and hill-climbs. Walking, in fact, is the wave of the future. Within a year or two, all those people who run just because someone told them they could lose weight or build stronger hearts will be striding across the planet, nodding and smiling at everyone they meet along their trails.

Walking is special. It's the only exercise that doesn't hurt. It's primarily an aerobic undertaking. It tones and limbers the lower-body muscles effortlessly and also tones your upper-body muscles if you concentrate on pumping your arms or use wrist weights. You can walk anytime, anyplace, in just about any clothing.

Walking is great for beginners. If you haven't exercised in years or if you're out of shape or have back problems, arthritis, high blood pressure, or heart trouble, you can start out walking slowly and pick up your pace when you're ready. Walking also provides a wonderful aerobic workout for even the fittest athletes. All they have to do is walk faster and faster or strap on some wrist weights or march up and down hills.

When you walk, even at a brisk pace, you have time to savor the world around you. "When I first started walking," Ellen Klein says, "I felt like a doddering old fool each time a runner blew past me. It's a good thing I was walking with a group. I don't know whether I would have been secure enough to walk by myself.

"But over the last two years, I've noticed a few things," she continues. "First of all, none of the runners smiles hello to me. Lots of walkers of all sorts—high school students coming home from school or shoppers on the way from the bus—nod and smile. Secondly, I still meet the exercise walkers I saw a year ago. The runners don't last more than a few months. Next, I often have long, gossipy chats with my friends as we march along. When you run, you can't talk. You're too winded."

Once you can walk a couple of miles, the world opens up to you. One day, you may wish to explore a neighborhood you've only whizzed past on the freeway. Another day, you may take a guided walking tour of the city's architectural or historical monuments. You may create your own museum tour: starting at the sculpture garden of one museum, then walking to the Rembrandt show in another museum a mile away. Some people love to walk completely unencumbered, feeling like birds blown by a breeze. Others prefer entertainment and don't mind carrying or wearing a tiny headphone-equipped tape player to listen to music or tape-recorded books.

## Buying and Testing Your Equipment

All you need is a good pair of shoes and you're off. A good walking shoe permits you to land on your heel, roll forward across the arch, and push off with your toes. Most running shoes work well for walking, although, technically, a walking shoe has a more flexible curved sole to allow your foot to bend across the ball of your foot as it rolls.

The choice in walking and running shoes is enormous. A knowledgeable sports shoe salesperson could guide you to the brands best for you, but you'll be lucky to find such a salesperson. The various walking and running magazines aren't much help either. The top-rated shoe in one magazine might very well sit at the bottom of the list in a rival magazine. Even experienced friends are little help. Every foot is different. The shoe flat-footed Frank touts as feeling as comfortable as a bedroom slipper is likely to be the very shoe that gives high-arched Helen cramps in every toe.

So, you'll have to go it alone. Here are the major things to look for.

A good shoe protects your foot from assault on several fronts. It has a moderately springy, cushioned sole that acts as a shock absorber, but it doesn't have to be as thick or springy as a running shoe because a walking stride doesn't create any impact forces on your feet. The sole and heel are wider than the shoe to keep you from twisting your ankle should you step into a pothole. The sole bends easily at the ball of the foot but has a stiff arch to keep your foot and ankle from wobbling from side to side inside the shoe. High-arched people need more support than flat-footed people. The toe box gives you enough room to wiggle and spread your toes a bit. There is about an inch of room between the end of your toes and the end of the shoe, because your foot moves forward inside the shoe when you walk, especially down even the slightest hill.

The heel counter (the stiffening material between the inner and outer layers of the shoe) fits snugly and is padded against your Achilles tendon. The inner sole has a cup to cradle the heel of your foot. The heel is rounded in the back so you don't stretch your Achilles tendon and pound your knees each time your heel touches the ground. The heel is somewhere between one-half and three-quarters of an inch high, close enough to the ground to give you some stability.

Fabric or leather shoes with mesh inserts over the toes permit sweat and heat to escape and so are cooler than solid leather in summer. However, they're sieves in rain and snow. Leather shoes, especially if waterproofed, keep your feet dry and warm in winter but are very warm in summer. Some new synthetic fabrics are waterproof yet breathe so your shoes don't turn into miniature sweat boxes.

When you try on new shoes, wear the socks you plan to exercise in. A shoe that fits over your thin argyles will probably feel tight over your thick sweat socks. Keep trying on shoes until you find one that feels almost as good as going barefoot.

Don't expect shoes to "break in." If they're not comfortable in the store, they never will be.

Run your hand inside the shoe to check for rough spots that will cause blisters. Look for a removable arch support. Should something happen to it, it's cheaper to replace the arch support than the whole shoe. Also, sometimes a shoe will fit comfortably if you throw away the factory-issued arch support and insert one of the several brands sold in sporting goods stores.

Place the shoes on a table and look at them from behind. If they lean to one side, they won't support your feet. Push down on the middle of the innersole with one finger. If the shoe rolls to the side, the shoe isn't properly engineered.

Many of the large chain department stores sell shoes with their own label for much less than the famous brand names. Often, the house-labeled shoes are made by one of those famous brand names—same shoe; the only difference is the label and the price.

Don't wear tennis shoes, racquetball shoes, aerobics shoes, or basketball shoes for walking, and don't wear walking shoes for any of those sports. Each shoe has its own type of toe box, arch support, last, ankle support, and traction. Aerobic dancing shoes, for example, are built for rocking from heel to toe, as walking and running shoes do, but they don't have enough traction for walking. Conversely, walking shoes have too much traction for aerobic dancing—you're likely to stop too suddenly in the middle of a dance move and twist your ankle or knee.

For those looking for entertainment or stimulation while they walk, the invention of the tiny portable Sony Walkman-style tape recorder was more important than the invention of the cushioned sweat sock. Some walkers go through several books on tape a year, listening to classics, murder mysteries, and how-to books. They study foreign languages. They filter out the urban frenzy by surrounding themselves with private music. They catch up on current events by listening to all-news radio stations. They borrow guide tapes (instead of guidebooks) from the public library about local wildlife and take mini-safaris around their neighborhoods. Book-taping companies advertise in most major magazines. Taped books are also available at chain bookstores and through large public libraries.

For mechanical treadmills for indoor walking, see Chapter 10.

# Clothing

In summer, dress as lightly as possible to avoid heat injury. Don't forget a sunscreen and a hat. You may not be running, but you'll still work up a sweat. In winter, dress in layers. Again, consider a sunscreen and wear your hat. If the temperature is under fifty or over seventy degrees, read Chapter 4 for information about protecting yourself against the weather.

# Warming Up

Warm up by walking slowly until you start to sweat and breathe a little harder. Then increase the pace to a nice aerobic huff-and-puff rate. Cool down by walking slowly for the last five minutes.

# The Basics

### FIVE-MINUTE LESSON

Before you start walking, drive prospective routes in your car to find out where one, two, three, and four miles end. After a while, you'll be able to tell how far you've walked just by your internal pace and the time elapsed.

For good walking form, first put one foot in front of the other. Next, put the other foot in front of the first. Come down on your heel, roll forward along the sole of your foot, and push off with your toes. Point your feet directly in front of you.

After you've walked fairly slowly for the first block or so to warm up your muscles and stimulate circulation, pick up the pace so you're walking as fast as you can comfortably. Walk fast enough to feel warm and to huff and puff a little, but you should still be able to talk to your companion or sing a song to yourself. (If you're not gently huffing, though, you're not getting a workout.)

If you're out of shape, start out on the flattest terrain you can find. If you must include hills, go uphill on your way out, and downhill on your way back home.

The first day, go slowly, even if it seems too easy. Don't just assume you can walk four miles. See what happens that first day. You probably won't feel sore while you walk, but if you're not used to exercising, you'll be giving your unused muscles a pretty good workout, and you may feel it later. If you don't ache that day, pick up the pace a bit the second day. If you do ache, continue to take it easy for a few more days.

During your first few days, walk just until you *begin* to feel tired, then turn around and walk back. Remember, you've got to walk as far to get home as you walked to get where you are.

As you walk, hold your head high, with good but not stiff posture. Good posture strengthens your abdominal and back muscles. Suck in your abdomen to strengthen them even more. Walk in a straight, purposeful, rhythmic, evenly paced gait. When you hit your stride, you'll feel weightless—it'll take no effort to keep moving.

What's fast for you may be slow to others, or vice versa. Work within your own capacity. Keep up this pace for twenty or thirty minutes at first but work up to forty-five minutes or an hour.

Don't stop along the way to window shop or talk with neighbors. You must walk *nonstop* for your constitutional to have the desired effect.

## SCHEDULE

Aim to walk three and a half to four miles in one hour at least three days a week—four, five, or six is better. If you haven't exercised for years, it may take you a few months to arrive at your goal. (Because walking doesn't strain your muscles the way some other sports do, it is one of the few sports you can do safely more than four times a week. That's one of the reasons people love it: they can walk off their worries every day, if they like, and enjoy the exhilaration of mild exercise without having to worry about overdoing.)

Once you've found your pace, experiment. Some people like to walk the same route every day because the walk seems shorter when they know exactly how far they've walked and how far they still have to go. Others get bored unless they change their routes frequently. Don't worry about how many miles you put in. If you walk at a huffing-and-puffing pace for forty-five minutes or an hour, you're getting a good workout.

## BEGINNER'S WALKING PROGRAM

*First week:* Walk until you *begin* to feel tired, then walk home. Try to walk at least five days a week.

*Second week:* Same. By now, you should be walking a little farther before you tire.

*Third week:* Same, but if you haven't increased your distance, do so now by adding two blocks this week, one at the beginning of the week and one at the end. (For you country folks, we're figuring a city block to be one-tenth of a mile, 176 yards. Therefore, two blocks is a little more than 350 yards.)

*Fourth week:* Same.

*Fifth week:* Add four blocks this week, two at the beginning and two at the end. If this feels too easy, add two more blocks at the end of the week. If it feels too hard, add only two blocks this week.

*Sixth week:* Same.

*Seventh week:* By now, you should be walking a mile and a half or two miles in forty to sixty minutes. From now on, add two to four blocks a week to your distance until you reach three or four miles. If you always walk at a brisk pace, your time per mile will go down as your mileage goes up, so you'll never be walking for much longer than an hour.

# Intermediate Walking

You are an intermediate walker if you walk four miles in one hour or less, at least four days a week. If you get to the point where the walk gets too easy—you're neither sweating much nor huffing and puffing—there are several ways you can intensify your workout.

First, pick up speed. Once you attain speeds of five miles per hour (twelve-minute miles) or more, it becomes harder to walk than to run and you expend much more energy on your walk.

Second, intensify your workout by lengthening your stride, raising your feet higher (as if you're marching), or exaggerating the swing of your arms. All of these take much more effort.

Third, carry weights. A half pound of weight strapped to

each wrist or carried in your hands (for a total of one extra pound) adds 5 percent (usually ten to twelve calories per hour) to your workout. That may not seem like much, but those twelve calories indicate that you're upping your aerobic workout. (Weights, of course, also strengthen your arms, shoulders, chest, stomach muscles, and legs.) You have several options for hand weights: a couple of cans of soda pop; water bottles filled with sand; plain cast-iron dumbbells; cloth-covered streamlined dumbbells with straps reaching across the back of your hand.

Our hands get tired from holding onto something for an hour. For that reason, we prefer to wear weights that encircle our wrists like heavy bracelets. Most wrist weights are fabric or plastic bands filled with lead pellets or sand and have Velcro closures to fasten them around the wrist. They work beautifully, but we much prefer the spongy, terry-cloth soft weights available in most sporting goods stores. You put these on as if you're shoving your hand through a doughnut and they conform to your wrist—no slapping around the way ordinary strap-on wrist weights do.

Seven pounds of weight strapped across your trunk bandolier-fashion adds the same twelve calories per hour to your workout. Some people wear backpacks or waist-belt affairs (often called fanny packs) filled with bags of sand or other unlumpy weights, but we don't advise either because they force your back to sway, and that could lead to a serious lower back injury. A loaded backpack also pulls back as you walk and bruises your armpits.

We don't recommend ankle weights. It's too easy to wreck your knees by wearing them.

Work yourself up slowly. Start out, if possible, with the half-pound wrist weights sold in aerobic dancing stores. Right there, you've added a pound. At first, the wrist weights will seem too light to do any good, but you'll discover that your legs get tired sooner. If you carry too much weight, you'll strain your knees, back, and even abdominal muscles. When the half-pound wrist weights seem too light, move up to one pound per wrist, and then two pounds. Eventually, if you get into very good shape, you can work yourself up to carrying about 7 percent of your body weight on your wrists, and that's quite a load. If you're using bandoliers, start with five or ten pounds and slowly work yourself up to about 10 percent of your body weight—for most of us—or 30 percent for the superfit. Or you can use a combination of wrist and bandoliers. Don't promote yourself too quickly. If you aren't ready for weights, you'll get cramps or pulled muscles.

# Masters Walking

You are a master walker if four times a week you walk four miles in fifty minutes or less while wearing two pounds of wrist weights (one pound per wrist) or fourteen pounds of bandolier weights.

If you want to further increase your workload, find some hills to climb. Walking up an 8.5-degree grade at 3.75 miles per hour—a real workout—should burn about 970 calories an hour for the average 150-pound man. (Note: 150-pound women, and people of either sex lighter than 150 pounds, burn fewer calories. People over 150 pounds burn more.)

Hill-climb first without weights. If this seems too easy, increase your pace and stride up every hill and down every valley you can find wearing weights, working yourself up to, say, twenty-five pounds in bandoliers and two-pound weights on each wrist. If you can do this, you're ready for the Olympics.

## SPEEDWALKING, OR RACE WALKING

Before you try out for the Olympics, try *speedwalking,* also called striding. Speedwalkers don't just enjoy their sport, they love it. Talk to people the day after they speedwalk their first three miles, and they're already singing rhapsodies. Talk to them two years later, and they've even more poetic. Once you discover speedwalking, whether you're twenty or sixty, you stick with it for life. It is stimulating and exhilarating yet unstressful. Says Angela Harmon, a forty-five-year-old high school French teacher and weekend speedwalking teacher: "Once you get the hang of speedwalking, the movements flow just like water. It's as if you're gliding downhill on skis and dancing at the same time."

Speedwalking is almost as good aerobic exercise as cross-country skiing and certainly holds its own compared with running or any of the other activities we describe. Top-notch

speedwalkers work themselves up to seven-minute miles—
many runners would kill for that pace—so this is no pantywaist
sport.

And yet it's very easy to learn and even easier to adjust to
your own pace. It's never too strenuous or too easy, it tones and
limbers both your upper and lower body, improves your posture and coordination, and burns, in the most highly trained
walkers, as many as 800 calories an hour. It's perfect for people
of all ages and is the only Olympic sport (under the *nom de
guerre* of race walking) that people over fifty have made their
own.

The only problem is that you look like an angry duck.
Speedwalking—also called aerobic walking, fitness walking,
power walking, health walking, exercise walking, dynamic
walking, or striding—is really just an exaggeration of plain old
ordinary fast walking. The technique is simple. As you take a
step, land on your heel and pull yourself forward as if you were
on a treadmill. Just as you're about to take another step, lock

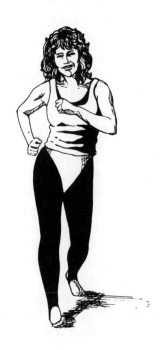

FIGURE 12.1 SPEEDWALKING.

your knee. Believe it or not, that's what you do every time you walk. It follows that whenever you completely straighten a leg, you stick your hip out (see Figure 12.1). At slow speeds, you're not aware of the hip swing, but at higher speeds, your hip really juts out to the side. It's natural and very comfortable (and loosens up your lower back even better than stretching like a cat). As you walk, pump your arms back and forth much more aggressively than you do with plain walking. Voilà! You're speedwalking.

All that twisting and turning sets the whole body atingle. The hip-swishing limbers up your hip and pelvic muscles; the arm-pumping loosens your shoulders and torso while it strengthens your arms and back; the gait strengthens and firms your legs; and the walking superconditions your heart and lungs. And it is still every bit as safe as regular walking.

Speedwalkers are unusually helpful folks. Just show up at a meeting of one of the local speedwalking clubs that have sprouted up around the country. The members are likely to greet you as if you were a long-lost cousin. When they learn you're a novice, they'll immediately offer more advice and helpful hints than you'll ever use.

Angela Harmon, for example, teaches speedwalking free of charge every Saturday and Sunday at meetings of her local racewalking club, where people of all ages show up. "I got into speedwalking by accident. I was taking a walk in the park, and there was this group of people standing around, so I went to see what it was about.

"It was a race walking meeting, and some of the members were explaining race walking to the beginners. I just joined in, and it was love at first sight. You don't have to be an athlete to race walk."

## ORIENTEERING

This combination of treasure hunt and footrace its you against the field or against yourself, depending on your preference. A national passion in Sweden, Australia, Japan, Israel, Switzerland, and some twenty other countries, orienteering teaches you to navigate over land using only a map and compass. Orienteering clubs throughout the country arrange weekly or monthly races through wooded parklands, and each one has easy, intermediate, and advanced courses.

Before each meet, members of the host orienteering club explain how to use a compass and how to read the topographical maps supplied by the club. The routes on the maps are color-coded by difficulty, the easiest ones following established trails, the more difficult ones requiring cross-country navigation. Over more difficult terrain, strategy is important because the most direct route may be unpassable due to hills or underbrush. Runners run, walkers walk, from one station to the next, punching their cards at each destination to prove they reached them all.

Orienteering is a competitive sport, but many people use the races as an excuse to get out into open country and go birdwatching instead. And, occasionally, fast walkers wipe out a field of runners because the walkers were shrewd enough to find much more efficient routes.

## HIKING AND TREKKING

Once you can walk four or five miles without stopping or feeling bushed, try longer walks—say a daylong hiking trip in any of several U.S. national parks. It's simple to plan these trips by yourself or with friends or family, but the hikes planned by local park districts, the Sierra Club, community centers, and church groups bring together people of similar age, condition, and interests and guide them along particularly interesting or little-known paths.

Many travel agencies sell walking trip packages (called treks) across the plains of Africa, through the foothills of Nepal, and around other storied countryside throughout the world. You walk at a moderate pace, usually with only a very light knapsack—if that much—while the tour transports your belongings, food, and other necessities from one meal stop to the next. Lodging is usually comfortably indoors, although camping out in fairly luxurious style is also an option.

# First Aid

You're not likely to get aches and pains from walking, and if something does happen, it's likely to be very mild.

**Aches down back of legs:** Stretch your hamstrings before and after each walk.

**Temporary sharp pains, cramps, or numbness in calf:** Stop and massage your calf. Stretch it by standing on the foot or by reaching down and pulling the toes upward. If that doesn't work, apply an ice pack for ten minutes. Prevent cramps by stretching before and after every walk, and by warming up your legs well before picking up speed. Cool down thoroughly, too. Wear shock-absorbing shoes. Eat potassium-rich foods (bananas, tomatoes, oranges, and potatoes) as well as foods rich in magnesium (peas, beans, nuts, green leafy vegetables) and in calcium (dairy products, broccoli, beans, oysters, turnip greens, mustard greens).

**Groin pain or any pain down the inside of thigh:** Apply ice pack or heat pack, whichever feels better. Stretch your hamstrings before and after each walk. Do groin stretches (see Chapter 3) during your cool-down. Check your shoes to see if they are unevenly worn down. Find out whether one leg is longer than the other. Even a quarter of an inch difference can cause enough of an imbalance and strain anywhere from your ankle to your back. You'll need the help of a friend for this. Lie down on the floor, on your back with your legs straight out in front of you. Using a tape measure, have your friend measure each leg from the center of your belly button to the top of your inner ankle bone. If one leg is longer than the other, put an innersole into the shoe of the shorter leg. Usually one innersole is enough, but if not, try two, as long as that doesn't make your shoe too tight.

**Shin splints:** If you develop a hot, searing pain or tenderness anywhere along the shinbone from ankle to knee, you probably have shin splints. See First Aid section in Chapter 11.

**Knee pain:** Most often caused by turning in your ankle or foot as you walk, called pronating. (It is also possible that your knee aches because you roll your ankle outward, but that's less common.) Having one leg shorter than the other also frequently causes knee pain. Other causes include spending too much time on your toes, very stiff muscles, very limber muscles, arthritis, and bursitis. See First Aid section in Chapter 11 for home treatment.

**Stabbing, searing, or dull pain in side or shoulder:** See First Aid section in Chapter 11 for more information on *stitches*.

**Blisters.** See First Aid section in Chapter 8.

If you asked us how to start exercising, we'd tell you to try walking first. No matter how unathletic you are, you can walk, so you'll start reaping aerobic rewards immediately. As your condition improves, you'll adjust the workload accordingly. Walkers are dedicated folks, not because they're fanatics, but because walking makes them feel so good. No wonder we call it the all-things-for-all-people sport.

# C H A P T E R   1 3

# This Is Not a Chapter About Running... Or Is It?

The running fad is done and gone. Most people new to exercise take up something else—usually walking—and the majority of those who do start running stop within six months. They throw their backs out. They hurt their knees. Or, once the novelty wears off, they realize how uncomfortable it is and how much they don't want to go out for their morning run. That's why more and more people are hanging up their running shoes and tying on their walking shoes.

It's about time.

## The Drawbacks

What do we have against running? A lot. All that hype a few years ago convinced a lot of people that running was the only decent aerobic exercise around. It's not. Running took on the aura of a new religion—if you converted to running, you would be saved from sloth, aging, pudginess, and heart disease. The

155

reward for the chosen was a "runner's high," a euphoric state pursued by many—often to ridiculous extremes of self-discipline and self-denial—but attained by only a small percentage of highly trained professional and semiprofessional long-distance runners.

So now it turns out that running isn't salvation. It's just a sport . . . one of many. It does have one distinction, though—it causes almost three-quarters of all the sports injuries seen by sports doctors: stress fractures of the feet and lower legs; shin splints; tears along the arch of the foot; heel spurs; inflamed Achilles tendons; ankle sprains; all kinds of knee trouble; disk injuries of the lower back; blisters; painful bleeding under toenails; stitches; excruciating pain in the ball of the foot; and serious heat injuries, to name but a few. If it weren't for running, most sports doctors would be out of business.

And these are just the injuries that strike healthy runners. What if you already have knee, neck, or lower back problems or arthritis or osteoporosis, or if you have certain types of heart disease, high blood pressure, or high blood cholesterol levels? Then running is even more dangerous.

To be fair, we have all heard of people who have used running, *under the guidance of their doctors,* to lower their blood pressure or serum cholesterol or to recover from some types of heart attacks. The fact is that running is indeed as beneficial as walking or swimming or any of the other aerobic exercises in this book for several types of cardiovascular conditions. But it's not *more* helpful. So why endure the discomfort and injuries running brings with it when you can do something else and get the same results?

Injuries are just one of our beefs against running. We consider running a threat to the public welfare because it turns so many people off exercise entirely. Only a few of us were born with the physical makeup to run day after day, week after week. The rest of us aren't built for it, mentally or physically. For us, running is more like a dose of cod-liver oil than a pleasant jaunt out in the sunshine. It takes a while, sometimes a long while (and sometimes never), before we're comfortable running. Usually, it's boring. And, for most of us, running never becomes a pleasurable activity. It just stays one giant pain. And pain for fun doesn't make much sense.

So, running gives exercise a bad name. People try running for a few months, realize they hate it, and swear off all exercise, even the easier and more healthful sports such as walking, cycling, or swimming—the ones they're likely to love stick with for the rest of their lives.

And running simply isn't aerobic enough for our tastes. Whenever you work as hard as you do running, you do some nonaerobic work, too. That means you put out all that effort but don't get quite as many health-giving aerobic rewards as when you walk, swim, row, cycle, or ski, indoors or out. In other words, running doesn't give you as big an aerobic return for your investment as most of the sports described in this book.

Running does strengthen your legs, especially the backs, but in the process it tightens your hamstrings and weakens the fronts of your thighs—unless, that is, you run up hills, and that's too strenuous for beginners. Because running tightens your hamstrings so much, you probably will have to stretch after each run to prevent muscle pulls. That adds time to your workout.

Running doesn't develop your upper body at all. Thus, if you want to firm up your trunk and arm muscles, you'll have to do something else in addition to running—swim, row, or ski, for example. You could, of course, wear wrist or bandolier weights or carry hand weights while you run, but these are also too strenuous for beginners. It's a whole lot easier to swim for aerobics in the first place, or walk with wrist weights, or row or ski indoors or out, and then you've got it all.

# A Joy for Some

Still, running is certainly one of the fastest ways of getting into good cardiovascular shape and losing weight. Running thirty minutes a day, three or four times a week, is all you need for optimal aerobic benefit. And there are those few people who are built for running. For them, running is a joy and a release. They are the people you meet who have been running five, ten, thirty years and have never hurt themselves. They're the ones who run ten miles on their birthdays to celebrate being alive. They're the ones who love the solitariness of running. They lose themselves in their own thoughts and in the rhythm of their strides. For them, running is an easy, natural, instinctive sport. They don't have to be taught how to run. They just go out and do it.

They're the minority. Still, it's possible that you happen to be one of those natural runners. If so, it would be a shame if you didn't discover your inborn talents. If you're curious about running, even after all these warnings, then try it. If you like it, if it makes you feel good, you're a runner. If you don't like it or if it hurts, slow down and thumb through the other chapters in this book to find your own ideal sport.

# The Basics of Running

First, check with your doctor if you have heart disease; high blood pressure; high blood cholesterol levels; knee, neck, or lower back problems; arthritis; or osteoporosis.

Then, start out with our Beginner's Walking Program (see Chapter 12). When you can walk three miles in forty-five minutes, buy yourself a pair of running shoes, the sort with a slightly less flexible, less curved sole than a walking shoe. (Be prepared, by the way, to replace your running shoes every two hundred miles or so. All that pounding breaks down the cushioning rubber and foam and cracks the outer covering. If you try to economize by wearing your old shoes too long, you'll wind up with foot and leg troubles galore.) Now you're ready to add a little jogging to your daily constitutional.

Warm up by walking. Then jog slowly for a minute, walk for a couple of minutes or as long as it takes to catch your breath, jog for another minute, walk for another two minutes, and so on for a half hour. Don't work too hard—keep everything at a nice even huffing-and-puffing aerobic level. In a couple of weeks, when this becomes easy, jog for a little longer —say one and a half or two minutes—then catch your breath by walking two minutes. When *this* feels comfortable, lengthen the jog again, but continue to alternate jogging and walking. Give yourself at least four months to work up to thirty minutes of nonstop jogging.

Never run two days in a row. Running is a strain, and your body needs a day off to recuperate. Run by the minute instead of the mile—thirty minutes at your own huff-and-puff level will give you all the aerobic rewards you want. Eventually you'll just naturally pick up speed but you won't feel the exertion.

Dress properly to avoid heat and cold injuries. Run in a straight line and keep your feet under your body. Breathe deeply through your mouth. Let your arms set the tempo for your stride the way they do when you walk. Relax your shoulders, bend your elbows, and swing your arms naturally back and forth. Step out with a comfortable stride. As your running becomes stronger, your stride will automatically lengthen a bit.

If you discover you like running, and if it makes you feel good, you'll want to perfect your technique, become adept in masters skills, and learn how to treat running injuries. *Galloway's Book on Running,* listed in the Resources section at the back of this book, should start you on the right road.

If you run thirty minutes straight, three or four times a week, you've found yourself a sport to last a lifetime. Thirty minutes is all you need for cardiovascular fitness, weight control, mental health, and all the other aerobic benefits. Since running more than thirty minutes a day or more than three or four times a week doubles your chances of hurting yourself, you have to love it to run more. If you love it that much, go to it . . . with our blessings.

# C H A P T E R 1 4

# Swimming:
# The Exercise That Does
# Just About Everything

**S**wimming is the most perfect movement there is. When you swim, the water holds you up the way an updraft supports a hawk. You glide through the water, smoothly, serenely, alone in your own private world, with just your thoughts and the incredibly cooling, refreshing, calming water around you. One woman says that swimming laps is like meditating. "I'm in a lovely, peaceful dream world," she says, "and I leave the pool renewed in body and spirit."

## The Pitch

Swimming does just about everything. It tones the muscles all over your body. It makes you more flexible, especially in the shoulders and ankles. It strengthens your heart and lungs effectively yet is very easy on the heart, because you move along horizontally on your stomach or back rather than vertically on your feet. The backstroke, in particular, relieves many types of back pain and may improve the hump-backed curvature that used to be called by the disgusting name "dowager's hump."

Swimming invigorates you without exhausting you. It keeps you cool in hot weather. (There is no one more smug than a swimmer, still damp from a morning dip, spying a walker or runner pouring sweat in the summer sun.)

One disadvantage is that swimming apparently doesn't increase bone mass (and, therefore, fight osteoporosis) because it doesn't force the bones and muscles to work against gravity.

Swimming helps you lose weight, but some researchers believe it's not quite as efficient a fat burner as dry-land exercises. Certainly, it will work off 95 percent of your excess fat, just as any other aerobic exercise will, but it may not burn off that last 5 percent. Explanation? Swimming in cool water (under eighty-five degrees) apparently triggers a blubber reflex in your body, causing your body to retain a *thin* outer layer of fat to insulate you and keep you warm. That 5 percent amounts to a couple of pounds—five if you're tall. Not worth worrying about unless you're applying for a job as a fashion model.

Swimming is the second most popular sport in the country, after walking, and for good reason. Anyone can swim. In fact, once you hit middle age, you (and overweight people of any age) have a special advantage over other swimmers: you float better because you have a higher percentage of body fat, and fat floats (like oil on water). That means you don't have to work as hard to stay on top of the water, and, therefore, you're a more efficient swimmer than you were in your twenties.

"All my life, I was terrified of the water," says Jason Trachtman, a fifty-year-old lawyer. "I grew up in a poor neighborhood and the only time I saw water was when someone turned on the fire hydrant.

"The older I got, the more it ate at me that I couldn't swim. So, on the day before my fiftieth birthday, I signed up for a beginning swimming class at the country club. I was nervous for the whole week before the class started.

"I was fortunate enough to have a terrific teacher who took things step by step, and in a few months, I was swimming eight laps a day, then sixteen, and now I've settled into twenty laps a day. It's a plus in my life. I love swimming. It gives me energy and a sense of accomplishment. And there's something about conquering a childhood fear. You go back to when you were eight and erase everything. And, you know, for the first time in my life, I look like a jock."

Since the turn of the century, doctors have recommended

swimming to fight the pain and stiffness of lower back problems and arthritis, especially arthritis of the knees. Its rhythmic, smooth motion stretches and strengthens joints and muscles and gives you easy, painless movement for hours afterward.

Over those years, swimming helped many, many people. However, there were always a few who got worse, not better, after swimming.

A few years ago, Ron had a patient who arrived suffering from excruciating back pain. She had been to four other doctors and none had been able to relieve the spasms that immobilized her for weeks at a time. Ron suggested, among other things, swimming, but she refused. Two other doctors had recommended the sport, but swimming was "a catastrophe," she said. "I was in pain for months."

"Try it my way," Ron said. "Swimming helps most people with back problems. Some do fine swimming the way they always have, but others get relief only if they don't overarch their backs when they swim. Some people who aren't good swimmers are afraid that their heads will sink into the water, so they arch their backs and stiffen their knees to keep their heads up. That makes their backs and knees hurt more, not less."

Ron convinced her to try his secret swimming weapon—a float belt. A float belt straps around your waist and is a grown-up version of the old inner tube around the middle. It keeps your trunk high in the water.

Ron's patient tried the float belt, and it worked wonders for her. Her back became stronger and more flexible and went into fewer spasms as the months went on.

The moral of the story? If you have back trouble, swimming will help. However, you'll have to experiment with and without the float belt to see which works best for you.

Float belts are sold in some swim supply shops, scuba dive shops, and even some kayaking and canoeing shops—including mail-order emporia—but they're hard to find because they are illegal in some states, including California. They are illegal to use as life preservers during any sort of boating because they aren't very buoyant and they don't keep your head out of the water. If you need a real life preserver, get one of the types suggested in Chapter 17. Float belts used as training devices for experienced swimmers in a pool violate no laws.

For people with back trouble, or people who aren't confident about swimming, we also recommend swimming with a snorkel and mask. This allows you to keep your head down in the water while you breathe continuously through the snorkel. This not only prevents the dreaded back overarch but also allows you to quit worrying about coordinating your swimming with your breathing.

**Don't swim without a doctor's approval if** you have epilepsy or have recently suffered a stroke (if you pass out or become disoriented, you could drown); or if you have recently had a mastectomy (your chest and underarm muscles may not be ready for the exertion); or if you have vertigo (an ear infection could aggravate it).

# Buying and Testing
# Your Equipment

For lap swimming, which is the focus of this chapter, look for a pool that sets aside special times for this activity. A pool crowded with children splashing water at one another is enough to turn anyone off. If you're in your forties or fifties, just about any decent lap pool will do, but as you enter your sixties and seventies, you'll need a pool heated to seventy-eight or eighty degrees, because you'll be more susceptible to the cold.

Many junior and senior high schools, community colleges, and universities open their pools to the public whenever school isn't in session. Large health clubs also offer lap swimming and water aerobics—some at reasonable prices. Private clubs are usually expensive, but they sometimes have cheaper monthly swimming-only rates. Community centers and Y's usually offer top-notch pool facilities and eminently reasonable prices.

If you have a pool, or a friend with a pool, you've got yourself a mixed blessing. Your pool gives you the ultimate convenience. However, the chances are your pool isn't twenty-five yards long. One woman told us she started swimming in her mother's ten-yard pool. "I got so I was swimming a mile in that little pool and my neck got so sore from turning that I had to find a larger pool."

# Clothing

Any swimsuit is fine as long as it stays up and as long as it doesn't rub or cut into your thighs or, for women, your shoulders, underarms, and back. A tight-fitting nylon cloth bathing cap will keep the hair out of your eyes without pulling it the way rubber caps do.

If your eyesight is so bad that you need glasses or contact lenses, ask your optician to put your prescription onto the new lightweight plastic watertight goggles that fit tightly around the eyeball. (These goggles, by the way, cured the water phobia of one of our friends. Although she knew the basics of swimming, she panicked every time she tried to swim more than five or six strokes in a row. One day, out of curiosity, she tried her grandson's goggles and easily swam the whole length of the pool. It turns out she wasn't afraid of the water. She was afraid of not being able to see.) One caution: Very tight goggles can cause headaches. Brands differ. Experiment to find a comfortable pair.

# Warming Up

You don't have to worry much about warming up until you start swimming a mile at a time. Just swim a few easy laps, then pick up speed. Cool down with a few more easy laps at the end of your swim. "Swimming is the only exercise I've ever done," says Janet Trachtman, restaurant owner and Jason's wife, "that feels wonderful the moment you begin. When you start running or even brisk walking, you've got to get your second wind before you feel good. When you start swimming, you stretch out and feel like you're being carried along by invisible hands."

# The Basics

### BEGINNING SWIMMING

If you already know how to swim, even if you haven't swum for thirty years, you don't need lessons. Just climb into the pool and start swimming laps. Your style and efficiency will improve if you stick with it, and within a week or two, you'll get to the point where you feel as if you could swim forever.

After a while, you'll probably want to take a class to learn the techniques that make so much difference. You may need help with your breathing, and a few lessons will help you swim faster and with much less effort. Or you may want to learn other strokes or drills to strengthen your kick.

If you can't swim at all, you will need lessons. You can't just get in there and paddle around enough to get any decent aerobic exercise. This is probably swimming's biggest drawback. Look for a teacher who specializes in teaching beginners or people who are afraid of the water. (Many beginners' swim classes cater to people who can already swim a little.) If you can't find a teacher, Cutherbertson and Cole's *I Can Swim, You Can Swim* is an excellent and instructive book (see Resources at the back of this book), but learning to swim from a book is a lot like learning to improvise jazz piano on a piece of black and white cardboard.

It's easy to learn to swim—even if you had trouble learning as a kid. Remember, you float more easily now. What's more, you can have the security of a float belt or mask and snorkel.

Swimming is easier on the circulatory system than walking, running, or any other upright, dry-land exercise. When you're lying down, as you do when you swim, your heart holds 10 to 20 percent more blood than when you're vertical. That means it pumps more blood with less effort during each contraction. Since swimming is less demanding and less jarring than most other exercises, after a while you'll have to put in a whole hour of swimming instead of the thirty minutes you can get away with in running. Also, if you want a good aerobic workout, you'll probably need four or five days a week, the way you do for walking, instead of three days for running. And you'll have to concentrate on working at a huffing-puffing pace because it's so easy to slack off while swimming.

For your daily swim, swim in a heated pool. You want that smooth water and the preset distance so you can pace yourself. (Save open-water swimming for paddling around with friends, and, when you do go to the beach, swim parallel to the shore within view of a lifeguard rather than pointing yourself straight out to sea.)

## FIVE-MINUTE LESSON

This five-minute lesson is for people who already can swim at least a little bit.

We recommend swimming with either the crawl (also called freestyle) or backstroke. They are the most efficient and beneficial strokes. Use the flutter kick, not the scissors kick, with the crawl. It's fine to use the breaststroke or the butterfly if you like, but they're more strenuous. In fact, use any stroke you enjoy as long as it's not the sidestroke, which works only one side of your body and is likely to lead to aches and pains along that side. What's more, it is the least effective for strengthening the heart. It's okay to use the side stroke for resting or cooling down, though the backstroke is even better for this. If you must swim the side stroke, learn to do it on both sides to keep everything balanced.

Swim in a straight line. Don't weave all over the pool because (1) you'll get in everyone else's way and (2) you'll wind up doing extra work. (The shortest route is a straight line.)

If you are swimming laps with other people, observe the lane markings and stay to the right side of your lane at all times. If you are a slow swimmer, use the outside lanes.

In the crawl, alternate breathing sides, coming up for breath one time on your left side, and then next time on your right. This not only makes the crawl a bilateral sport but also keeps you swimming in a straight line.

Coordinating your breathing with your stroking is one of the trickiest parts of swimming. Let the air trickle from both your nose and mouth at first, but explosively blow the last bit of air out into the water just as you start tilting your head out of the water for the next breath. This clears the water away from your mouth so you can take a fresh breath more easily. Most accomplished distance swimmers breathe once for every pair of left-right strokes.

In the crawl and butterfly, keep your elbows high. Begin your arm pull with your elbow almost straight; then, about halfway through the stroke, bend your elbow a little more than ninety degrees in order to push the water back forcefully.

Keep your body as straight and flat as possible. Lightly point your toes, submerge your face to your hairline, and keep your legs high. All this streamlines you into a humanoid torpedo. Don't bring your feet to the surface or you'll be kicking air.

Don't wiggle or roll from side to side or you'll become more like an empty barrel than a streamlined torpedo.

If you get bored with plain old swimming strokes, try using hand paddles or kick boards for a few laps each day. Not only will they add variety to your workout but they'll also strengthen your strokes and kicks.

## SCHEDULE

At first, you probably won't be able to swim a single length all the way through. That's all right. When you get tired, grab the side until you catch your breath, then start again. Keep up this start-and-rest system for as long as you need it. Each day, you'll be able to go farther, and soon you'll be swimming several laps nonstop. (A lap is two lengths of the pool—up and back.)

The idea is to work yourself up, over a period of weeks or months, to sixty minutes of nonstop, slightly huffing swimming. That will probably settle down to 800 or 1,000 yards, thirty-two to forty lengths in a 25-yard pool. If that sounds like a lot at first, just do what you can. Soon, you'll find that you just don't want to get out of the pool. It feels too good. You'll become absorbed in the rhythm of your strokes, the regular beat of your kicks, and the soothing comfort of the water. (See Beginner's Swimming Program on the following page.)

# Intermediate Swimming

As a general rule, don't worry about your time when you swim. As long as you're huffing and puffing, you will automatically swim faster and farther as your stamina improves.

However, when you think you're ready to move out of the beginners' ranks and into more intensive training, time yourself against the large pace clock that hangs on one wall of every serious lap pool.

You are an intermediate swimmer if: you are forty to sixty years old and can swim 100 yards in less than two and a half minutes and 1,000 yards in less than twenty-five minutes; or if you are over sixty and can swim 100 yards in three minutes and 1,000 yards in twenty-seven to thirty-two minutes, depending on how much over sixty you are. (Unless you're in very good

## BEGINNER'S SWIMMING PROGRAM

| WEEK | PROGRAM | NONSTOP DISTANCE |
|------|---------|------------------|
| 1 and 2 | 100 yards, divided into four parts, each of 25 yards, with a rest period between each | 25 yards |
| 3 through 5 | 200 yards, divided in half (100 each); rest between each | 100 yards |
| 6 through 15 | 400 yards, divided into four parts (100 each); rest between each | 100 yards |
| 16 through 23 | 600 yards, divided into three parts (200 each); rest between each | 200 yards |
| 24 through 31 | 800 yards, divided into four parts (200 each); rest between each | 200 yards |
| 32 through 40 | 800 yards, divided into two parts (400 each); rest between each | 400 yards |
| 40 | 800 yards nonstop | 800 yards |

If this schedule moves too slowly for you, move on to the next stage sooner. If it moves too briskly, stay at each stage longer.

---

shape, you lose about 1 percent of your speed each year after your sixtieth birthday.)

From now on, swim a bit faster, knocking seconds, then minutes, off your time. Add yardage whenever you fall below the forty-five or sixty minutes you allot to your swimming workout.

For variety and an even better workout, swim intervals once or twice a week instead of long, steady distances. To swim intervals, speed up and slow down every few minutes. Begin with a slow warm-up speed for five minutes; then swim 400 yards at a fast pace; then slow down to a moderate pace for another five minutes; then swim at top speed for a length or two; then swim at a moderate pace for another five minutes; and so on for the hour. Never swim so fast, however, that you have to stop to catch your breath.

If you want to strengthen your strokes, immobilize your legs (and your kick) by sticking them into styrofoam "floats" or "pull tubes" made of rubber tubing; then swim a lap or so. Or develop your arms by working out with hand paddles or webbed swim gloves. To strengthen your kick, don't stroke. Instead, hold onto a kickboard and flutter-kick your way up and down the pool. These training aids are best used under the tutelage of a coach.

# Masters Swimming

You are a master swimmer if you can swim 3,500 yards (or two miles) nonstop. That is beyond most of us, and that's just as well, because it's the advanced swimmer who's likely to get hit by swimmer's shoulder, cramps, and breaststroker's knee.

If you're the competitive type, swimming has the best organized masters programs in the country. Masters programs are races organized for people over the usual competitive age in any given sport. Each organization has its own entrance requirements. For example, since most competitive swimmers are over the hill at nineteen, U.S. Masters Swimming begins with nineteen-year-olds. However, you must be forty or over to enter a Masters Swimming Program race.

In masters meets, each event is age graded; you swim only against people within five years of your age. Swim meets include 100-, 200-, and 400-yard races in each of the competitive strokes (freestyle, butterfly, backstroke, and breaststroke), as well as medleys and long events of 1,650 yards (1,500 meters).

"Masters races may be the only place where people get prizes for getting older," says Felix Tejada, a forty-six-year-old butterfly racer (and welder in his off-swimming hours). "I know a sixty-nine-year-old woman—a freestyle swimmer—and she can't wait until her seventieth birthday. Then she moves up a division, but since she'll be the youngest in the seventy to seventy-fours, she'll clean up."

Why does Felix race? "It makes me feel younger. I prove to everyone that I'm not over the hill. It shows I can hang in there with the best of them."

Although we define a master swimmer as someone who can swim two miles nonstop, most masters races don't require that level of expertise. In some divisions and some distances, an intermediate swimmer may have a good chance of winning a medal. Most public pools have their own masters swim clubs or keep a list of nearby swim teams. Or contact U.S. Masters Swimming, Masters Swimming Program, and Senior Olympics (see Resources at back of this book) for swim clubs and races in your area.

# Other Swimming Activities

There's more to swimming than laps in a pool. Consider some of these alternatives.

## AQUAEROBICS

How about aerobic dancing in water? Sound too easy? Don't count on it. You don't know what hard work is until you try running in deep water while wearing a flotation vest to keep you upright.

Aquaerobics is also called water aerobics or aquatic exercise. Most YMCAs and health clubs offer daily or weekly classes. They are usually organized similarly to aerobic dance classes, graded into beginning, intermediate, and advanced and require you to take your pulse frequently to keep your heart rate in a target range. Aquaerobics is a godsend for people with bad knees, bad backs, arthritis, or any other problem that eliminates landlocked exercise, but it is super exercise for anyone.

Classes can be a combination of dancelike routines, calisthenics, swimming strokes, actual swimming, and synchronized swimming—some or all of the above. Some use music. The principle is simple: the water resists your movement so you get a safe, exhilarating workout without any bone-crushing strain or jarring.

If you can't find a class nearby—or if you're lucky enough to have a pool and don't want to leave home—follow the routines in Jane Katz's *The W.E.T. Workout* (see Resources). It's up to you to figure out how to read the instructions in the pool.

## WATER POLO

How about water polo, one of the most strenuous sports in the world? It takes power, flexibility, stamina, coordination, and a good sense of strategy—a wet combination of basketball, swimming, and ice hockey. Not every pool fields a water polo team. You may have to ask around, or write the Master's Swimming Program, U.S. Masters Swimming, or the Amateur Athletic Union, Water Polo section (see Resources).

## SYNCHRONIZED SWIMMING

Synchronized swimming is every bit as demanding but doesn't involve the rough body contact of water polo. Forget Esther Williams breaststroking through a pool of flowers while twenty sweet young things dive in at one-second intervals. Today's synchronized swimming is a tough sport demonstrated for the first time in the 1984 Los Angeles Olympics. If you don't believe it, just try doing an upside-down corkscrew spin in slow motion with your head down in the water and your legs and hips completely above the water. Contact the Masters Swimming Program, U.S. Masters Swimming, or the National Institute for Creative Aquatics (see Resources).

## SNORKELING AND SCUBA DIVING

Snorkeling is a snap to learn in a few minutes from a good teacher. Scuba diving, however, takes weeks and months of professional lessons but is worth every minute. Talk about seeing the world! You see hundreds of worlds, glorious worlds under the waters of Australia, Guam, Hawaii (except for the area around Waikiki), the Bahamas—anywhere the ocean is still full of living corals, sea plants, and wild life —colors and shapes that exist nowhere else. Most hotels near good snorkeling beaches offer snorkeling gear for rent and will arrange lessons from a reliable snorkeling teacher. Scuba diving lessons are available through universities and dive shops listed in the Yellow Pages. Make sure your instructor has been trained and certified by the National Association of Underwater Instructors, the Professional Association of Diving Instructors, the YMCA, or the Los Angeles County Department of Parks and Recreation. These four organizations have the oldest and most rigorous training programs in the country.

# First Aid

Swimming rarely causes injury. When you begin swimming, you may experience some pain in your shoulder, but that should disappear after a few days.

**Swimmer's shoulder:** Shoulder pain after you've been swimming a few months indicates swimmer's shoulder, caused by overusing or using incorrectly the muscles in your upper arm, chest, and shoulder.

Apply an ice pack for ten minutes every few hours for a day or two. Try some or all of the following suggestions: Stretch your shoulder, chest, and upper back muscles before and after every swim. Keep your shoulders loose by rolling them backward and forward a few times a day. Ask yourself if you've been overdoing it, and if the answer is yes, back off. If the answer is no, perhaps the fault lies in your stroke. Don't bring your stroking arm too far across your body. Instead, roll your body toward your arm as it strokes through the water. If the pain is in your dominant arm, alternate sides as you breathe. The arm on the breathing side always works harder.

**Stabbing, searing, or dull pain in shoulder, neck, or side:** See First Aid section in Chapter 11 for information on *stitches.*

**Irritated, red eyes:** Wear goggles to keep the acidic, chlorinated water out of your eyes. The burning should go away within a couple of hours.

**Bloodshot eyes:** Blame it on the goggles. When you surface dive in the deep end of the pool, the deep water exerts pressure on the air inside your goggles, and that pressure pops the tiny blood vessels in your eye. It probably doesn't do any long-term damage, but to prevent it you have a few choices, none of them perfect. First, don't dive. Second, don't wear goggles when you dive. Third, wear a face mask when you dive because the passage between your nose and your lungs equalizes some of the pressure inside the mask, thus reducing the pressure on your eyes. Fourth, try wearing smaller goggles. Smaller goggles mean smaller air space, which means less air pressure. However, smaller goggles may also mean goggle headaches (see below).

**Headaches while swimming or immediately afterward:** May be caused by tight goggles or by goggles that fit too snugly into the soft flesh around your eyeball. Experiment with other brands.

**Itchy skin:** Usually comes from chlorine. Shower thoroughly in fresh water as soon as you get out of the pool.

**Painful sinuses, sinus headaches, or sinus infections:** Wear nose clips when you swim.

**Hair dries out, changes color, or gets tangled easily:** Wet your hair in the shower or sink before swimming, towel-dry away the drips, then apply a tiny bit of light conditioner or cream rinse to your hair before putting on your bathing cap. The rinse or conditioner traps the moisture inside your hair so it can't absorb any in the pool. Wear a waterproof cap with a Velcro band for as leakproof a seal as possible. Afterward, in the shower, rinse out the cream rinse, then massage a rinse designed to strip medication film, trace minerals, and metal residues from your hair. Let this stuff sit in your hair while you wash the chlorine off the rest of your body; then rinse out the stripper, shampoo as usual, and if your hair seems dry, use a conditioner.

**Oozing, itching, or aching ear(s):** The famous swimmer's ear is caused by continuous dampness in the ear canal. Each day, carefully dry your ear with cotton swabs, then apply the merest bit of rubbing alcohol with clean, dry swabs. (Don't stick the swabs into your ear.) Experiment with ear plugs. Some of the latest models don't just fit inside the ear canal but cover the entire ear. Ask your local sports medicine clinic or swim coach for a local source.

**Colds:** To avoid catching cold during the winter, dry your hair before you go outside, and wear a hat or scarf.

**Heat exhaustion:** Believe it or not, you can suffer heat exhaustion even in a cool swimming pool. Although the water cools your body, you still sweat a great deal. Therefore, drink as much water as you can before and after each workout.

Because swimmers work out in a private world, with little contact with other people or the noise and bustle of reality, they get a bonus of calming meditation every time they exercise for fitness and good health. No wonder most of the famous swimmers from earlier Olympics and the movies have lived into their seventies and eighties—Johnny Weismuller, Buster Crabbe, Esther Williams, just for starters—and many of them are still going strong. Swimming, indeed, is more than just wonderful exercise. It's the ultimate escape and the perfect relaxation.

# CHAPTER 15

# Cycling:
# Getting There Is More
# Than Half the Fun

**L**ots of my friends use their bikes for transportation," James Wang told us one day, "and lots of my friends ride bikes for fun, but I'm the only one I know whose life was changed by his bicycle."

Wang, a television producer in San Diego, recently celebrated his sixtieth birthday by making a 100-mile tour with sixty of his closest pals in his bicycle club. At the end of the ride, he treated them all to a Chinese banquet.

"When I turned fifty, it meant the end of all hope. I was sure there was nothing left for me. I'd never be a boy wonder again, and all those young kids were breathing down my back. I was afraid I was going to lose my job.

"I was about fifty pounds overweight. I had terrible back pains and every few months I'd be flat on my back for two or three weeks. I felt old. Really old.

"One day my son, who was working up to a European bike tour, talked me into taking a ride with him, but it was a disaster. I couldn't keep up with him. The smallest hill killed me. I didn't know how to use the gears. I stopped after about fifteen minutes and sat on the side of the road for an hour and waited for my son to come back to get me.

"I'm not sure why, but a few days later, I got out my daughter's bike and tried it again. I didn't get any farther, but it didn't seem so hard because I was alone and I could slow down whenever I needed to.

"After that, I got to liking it. I rode many times a week. After a few months, I bought my own bike—a mountain bike with fat tires. I hate skinny tires like on my daughter's touring bike. They rattle your bones. My bike's also got a much more comfortable seat, and you sit upright instead of hunched over.

"Then my wife died. After a while, I had to get out and be with people, so I signed up for a weekend desert bike tour through our church. It had its ups and downs, but overall, it was great to get away and it was great to see the desert close up.

"The leader of that trip belonged to a bicycle club. This club was started at the end of the last century and is still going strong. Its five hundred members—some in their twenties and some in their eighties—ride together every day and take special rides every weekend. He sort of pushed me into going on a ride with them that next weekend.

"That was more than eight years ago. Now, I ride with the club four or five days a week. I see many of those people more than I see my family or the people I work with. The club saw me through a bad period, and it became a mirror that reflected my whole life."

# The Pitch

It's no coincidence that the James Wangs of the world are drawn to bicycling. Bicycles are so efficient, they do 30 percent of the work for you. You don't have to overtax yourself as a beginner. You sail along enjoying the scenery, with the wind ruffling your hair and the breeze cooling your skin, and, all of a sudden, you've eaten up ten miles—much more than you could cover if you were running or walking. And you barely felt it.

And yet, as you get stronger, your workout keeps pace— you go faster and farther, climbing a few hills here and there, and you get just about all the aerobic exercise you need.

Then, for those drawn to this sort of thing, there's the fascination of all that gadgetry. You've got that great big toy —a lovely, gleaming machine—with brakes to squeeze, gears to shift, chrome to polish. Also, you've got skills to experiment with. What happens if I lean this way? What if I try an easier gear? How tightly can I steer around that manhole cover?

With cycling, the novelty doesn't wear off, because you can always distract yourself with all sorts of accessories: rear-view mirrors, cycling shoes, seat covers, maybe even a brand-new, fancier bike.

Cycling has a lower drop-out rate than running or swimming, and one of the reasons is that once you've made this kind of financial commitment, you're more likely to stick with it. Even if you bought a very well-used bike from a neighbor for only a few bucks, it seems a shame to throw away that money.

By the way, there's more to cycling than two wheels. That's why this chapter is titled Cycling, not *Bi*cycling. For instance, a new species, the adult tricycle, handles like a good bike and rides like a Cadillac. It's the perfect solution for people who have slightly impaired balance or who can't get the hang of riding a two-wheeler.

Right now, trikes are most popular with the over-sixty crowd. Quadricycles, however, are the high-tech babies of some of the most ingenious inventors in America today. When these superefficient quadrikes escape the inventor's workshop and enter the world of mass production and competitive pricing, we predict they'll become the transportation of choice for short-haul trips.

Cycles of all sorts have a special advantage over other forms of exercise—they provide practical transportation. "Lots of people in our club commute on their bikes every day," James Wang says. "Of course, we live in a warm climate. We never have to worry about snow or ice. Still, if I lived out east, I'd ride during the nice seasons, take my bike grocery shopping, that sort of thing. An expensive bike costs one-twentieth of a car, doesn't need any gas or insurance, and is easy to park."

All this and health too. Cycling strengthens your heart and lungs and gives you all the aerobic benefits. It tones up all of your muscles from the hips down, especially the front of your thighs, though it does almost nothing for your upper-body muscles. A properly adjusted bike gives you a stress-free ride. Your legs move in smooth, flowing arcs—no bouncing or jostling—and the seat supports your weight. That's why many doctors recommend cycling to overweight people (no jiggling) and to patients recovering from heart attacks.

**Don't cycle without a doctor's approval** if you have Ménière's disease or other sorts of dizziness (your bad balance and the bike's bad balance are a bad combination); or if you have chronic back trouble.

# Buying and Testing Your Equipment

A bike is a relatively expensive purchase. We recommend borrowing a bike or buying a very cheap used one until you know for sure that you like cycling.

Should you choose to buy a bike, you'll have a number of decisions to make. First, bicycles come in three frame styles: what we used to call "men's" and now call "standard"; what we still call "women's"; and what everyone spells *mixte* but pronounces "meext" if they're French and "mixty" if they're American. It means—you guessed it—mixed or hybrid.

Women's bike frames are cut low; you just step across them to get on the seat. Unfortunately, this convenient design is weak and wobbly. Men's frames have that high bar from under the seat across to the post holding the handlebars. To mount the bike, you have to swing your leg back and over the seat to reach the opposite pedal. This requires a good measure of flexibility in your hips. However, this frame is very sturdy. Mixte combines the virtues of the other two frames. Its top bar is low enough to half-step/half-swing across, but high enough to reinforce the frame.

Second, you have to find a cycle that's scaled to your height and the length of your legs. Bikes and trikes come in several sizes. They used to be measured by wheel size. Now they are measured by frame size, which means the distance from point A, where the seat post slides into the frame, to point B, the center of the crank (the long shaft with the pedal on one end and the axle on the other).

When you're seated on the cycle, both feet should *just* touch the ground. Your leg should be slightly bent when your foot reaches the bottom of the pedal stroke. If it's bent a lot, the cycle is too small and you'll hurt your knees pedaling.

When you're straddling the cycle, the crossbar on a standard bike should come almost to your crotch, but not quite.

Third, you've got to decide what posture you want to ride in. Cycles come in bent-over (racer's crouch), upright riding, and recumbent models. On an upright, you sit as if you were sitting on a dining room chair. On a racer's crouch model, you bend forward in a tuck, as if you were kneeling in the starting blocks for the Olympic 100-meter footrace. Even the sturdiest backs and necks ache after a few minutes in that crouch; your hands get sore on those dropped, ram's-horn handlebars; and, worst of all, you can't see where you're going. We don't see much purpose to bent-over riding unless you ride more than thirty miles a day nonstop and are terribly worried about being aerodynamically streamlined. On a recumbent, you ride leaning back as if you were reclining in an easy chair with your feet on an ottoman. It takes a few minutes of practice to learn to balance and judge distances on these new reclining bicycles, tricycles, and quadricycles, but once you get the hang of it, you'll discover that pedaling is much easier. And that's the whole point. Recliners work on the same principle you use when you want to push a very heavy box: you get down on the floor, wedge your back against the wall, and push with your legs, using all of the forward power of your large thigh muscles, the largest and strongest muscles in your body.

Recumbents make good sense, but they're hard to find and cost a bundle. So, overall, upright wins the day. More and more serious cyclists are trading in their old drop-handled touring and racing bikes for new mountain bikes and other upright models. They're much more fun to ride.

Fourth, decide whether you want skinny or fat tires. Bikes with skinny tires are difficult to balance and give a hard, bumpy ride. Bikes with wide, balloon-style tires ride soft and easy and grip the road better.

Fifth, you have a wide choice of gearing—too wide. No-speeds, such as the old Schwinns many of us rode as kids, have foot brakes and are fine for flat terrain. If you've got even the slightest of hills in your neighborhood, however, you're better off with a three-speed (or three gear setting) bike or trike. Shifting from one gear to another cuts in half the effort you exert pedaling uphill, just as shifting from a higher to lower gear gives your car more power up a hill. Three-speeds come with either foot or hand brakes.

Most people don't need more than three-speeds. In fact, most people with ten-speeds use only three speeds (or gears). However, if you live in a decidedly hilly area, or if you just plain enjoy tinkering with gadgetry, a ten-speed bike or trike will definitely make your rides easier. For street riding, forget the twelve- and fifteen-speed bikes. They're mainly for off-road explorations through mountainous dirt paths and underbrush. Whatever the gearing, make sure the gearshift lever is conveniently placed on the handlebar, not down between your legs.

If you opt for an upright, wide-tired, hand-braked, ten-or-more speed, standard-style bike, consider the mountain bike, the rage of the eighties. Yes, it eats up mountains, but it's just as light, smooth, and easy to handle on a city street. It weighs little more than skinny-tired ten-speeds and yet it's three times as sturdy—you're not as likely to fold up a tire rim by riding over a curb as you are on a skinny-tired job. The tires themselves turn the roughest road into a mattress-soft path and yet are almost impossible to puncture. They're a lot like riding your old Schwinn but with reliable hand brakes and fifteen or more gears—unnecessary for most city riding, but the bikes don't come any other way, and you'll love them if you ever try any off-road riding. (Names for these bikes vary in various parts of the country: "mountain bike," "cruiser," "klunker," "off-road bike," "wilderness touring bike," "all-terrain bike," and "lightweight fat-tired bike.")

If you have a dedicated riding partner and a few extra bucks to spare, look into tandems. They are as sleek as any other ten-speed, go a lot faster (forty miles an hour isn't unusual), feel solid on the bumpiest roads, and permit you to conduct conversations without shouting. If you can't afford a tandem, try Instant Tandem, a gadget that links two standard bikes together to make one fairly well-designed tandem.

Other equipment? People who ride long distances swear by toe clips, which are tiny cages bolted over the front of each pedal. You slip your feet into the clips and voilà! You do twice the work with half the energy: as you *push* down on one pedal, you *pull* up the other. Toe clips protect your knees and thighs from the aches and pains of overuse, but—and this is a big but—they are dangerous. Once you get your feet into them, it's very hard to get them out. If you feel you're falling, you may not be able to put your foot down in time to check your fall.

Seats (or saddles) come in wide and narrow, soft and hard, leather and plastic. Wide saddles are much more comfortable but often rub your inner thighs raw and may cause knee problems on long rides because they push your legs too far apart. Narrow saddles are hard and uncomfortable—it takes at least a month for a saddle to break in your anatomy—but they keep your legs together and spare the knees. Leather absorbs sweat, plastic rides hot. Chamois seat covers absorb even more sweat and feel velvety. Many cyclists swear by sheepskin seat covers. They not only absorb sweat but also soak up bumps and are luxuriously comfortable. They're expensive, though. We prefer a rubbery foam seat cover (made of the same material as innersoles). It absorbs perspiration and cushions your fanny better than just about anything else on the market. It's also the most expensive.

Two words about cycling helmets: Wear them. And put them on your children. In bicycling accidents, even minor ones, the head and face are injured more often than any other part of the body. A good helmet improves your chances of avoiding such injury by 50 percent. With helmets, you get what you pay for. Buy one of the hard-shell types with ventilation holes and good shock-absorbing foam inside. It should be light and shouldn't obstruct your forward or peripheral vision. Make sure it doesn't have big gaps through which you could be impaled. If you do get into an accident in which the helmet absorbs a blow, throw it away and buy another. When the polystyrene foam padding cushions your head against a heavy blow, it is compressed and never bounces back completely to its original resilience. Make sure that whatever helmet you buy *meets or surpasses* the American National Standards Institute's specifications.

Rearview mirrors that attach to your handlebars give you eyes in the back of your head. We prefer these to the little dental mirrors mounted on helmets or eyeglasses, because handlebar-mounted mirrors have a larger field of vision. With helmet or eyeglass mirrors, you have to tilt or nod your head to focus behind you. We also prefer permanently mounted rearview mirrors to wrist or glove mirrors. With a wrist or glove mirror, your field of vision changes every time you move your hand. Rearview mirrors do have two flaws. First, because they're mounted on your handlebars, they focus on someone's front lawn—instead of on the traffic behind you—every time you round a corner. Second, you have to take your brake assembly apart to install the mirror.

Toys, toys, toys. Want still more fun? Attach a bicycle computer to measure your speed and distance. The little read-out box mounts on your handlebars and connects to one or more magnets attached to the front wheel. Prices for these are falling but now hover around thirty to seventy dollars. Some computers also measure cadence (the number of pedal revolutions per minute) and include a stopwatch, alarm, and countdown, but these features are unnecessary unless you don't wear a watch. Price is not an indication of quality. Test each model to make certain it records your current speed instantly (some lag several seconds behind or go haywire from ghost vibrations of the magnets). As a general rule, the more magnets, the faster and more accurate the computer. On good computer models, you reset the trip meter simply by pushing a button. On poorly designed computers, you have to remove and reinsert the batteries in order to reset the meter.

If you use your bike for commuting, touring, or shopping, you'll need some combination of saddlebags, panniers, or other sorts of baskets to carry your briefcase, luggage, and groceries. The array is endless, including some that collapse out of the way when not in use. Try to find a size that holds a loaded grocery bag. It's a pain to have to unpack your groceries on the sidewalk and repack them, piece by piece, into your saddlebags.

See Chapter 7 for indoor exercise bikes or wind trainers. (Wind trainers turn your own bike into an exerciser. They are vastly easier to use than the tricky "rollers" or other racing mounts used by athletes in training.)

# Clothing

Wear any sort of clothing as long as nothing can get caught in the chain or wheel spokes. Fifty-cent pants clips keep slacks from flapping around and getting into your chains.

Even in relatively mild weather, you may get chilled because you create your own wind-chill factor when you ride (see Table 4.2, wind-chill factor chart). For example, if the thermometer reads forty-five degrees Fahrenheit outside, the wind is blowing at ten miles per hour, and you're riding at fifteen miles per hour, the wind and you make a combined wind speed of twenty-five miles per hour. At this wind speed, forty-five degrees on the thermometer feels like twenty-three degrees on the skin, which is pretty cool. That cold, combined with the fact that you're wet from sweat, could lead to hypothermia. When the air temperature is above forty-five or fifty degrees, you can dress in layers and stay warm enough. Below that, it's time to go indoors.

Even in relatively mild weather, expect your hands and feet to get cold. Wear polypropylene gloves available from camping stores. Polypro is warm but thin so you can still operate brake levers and gearshifts. If it's not too cold, cut the finger tips from one pair for better dexterity with brakes and gears. For the feet, polypro socks or a combination of silk sock liners and polypro socks can't be beat. Dress for your wind-chill factor, not the temperature. See Chapter 4 for more information on dressing for the weather.

# The Basics

## FIVE-MINUTE LESSON

If you rode a bike as a kid, you'll probably find it easy to pick up again. Your balance will probably come back very quickly. Getting the hang of hand brakes may be a little harder. Those of us used to childhood coaster (foot) brakes instinctively try to backpedal every time there's an emergency stop. The panic this can cause lasts for only a few rides and then the hand brakes seem more sensible. (They grab more quickly and more precisely.) Learning how to shift gears takes much longer, but all the time you're learning, you're riding.

If you've never ridden a bike before, you'll feel like a six-year-old all over again. You have two choices: accompanied or solo. Accompanied requires one generous, patient friend. You pedal slowly—trying to figure out how to pedal and keep the bike straight at the same time—while the helper runs along beside the bike, holding onto the seat and doing most of the work of keeping the bicycle more or less upright for you.

Solo is easier on the ego but takes a little longer. First, temporarily lower the seat so your feet scoot along the ground.

Push yourself off with your feet to get a rolling start, lift your feet from the ground, and try to balance. If you tip to the side, put your foot down to catch yourself. When you're comfortable with this balancing act, put your feet up on the pedals and start gently pedaling. You'll be going a little faster but that actually makes balancing easier, not harder. When you can ride without putting your feet down every few seconds, return your seat to its proper height and keep practicing.

Alternately, you can just buy yourself a tricycle and hop on. No lessons and very little practice are necessary.

Once you get the hang of staying on the bike and keeping it rolling, consider these pointers:

- At first, ride on the flattest terrain possible. Uphill is hard work. Downhill, even the smallest downhill, feels like a plunge down a roller coaster. Don't ride in rain or snow—the roads are too slick. Move indoors to an exercise bike or wind trainer (see Chapter 7).
- Ride in a straight line without wobbling or swerving.
- Shift without taking your eyes off the road.
- Lean a bit into turns.
- Don't swerve your bike when you turn your body to look behind.
- Practice tight turns around potholes or broken glass in the street. This is one of the best indicators of how well you control your bike. Ideally, your front wheel passes to one side of the obstacle while your rear wheel takes the other side.

## SCHEDULE

Your first goal is to ride thirty minutes nonstop at a decent pace. This will probably take you six months or more to achieve. Start by cycling only until your legs *begin* to feel tired. Then cycle back home. Ride at a *mildly* huffing-puffing pace. Cycling is hard on the thighs, and if you pedal up a good sweat, your legs will give out before you get a good aerobic workout. Ride in a medium gear—just enough to put in some moderate effort—on flat terrain.

## CYCLING SAFETY TIPS

Cycling injuries have become a national epidemic ever since we started riding on the streets instead of the sidewalks. To protect yourself, think of yourself as just another car on the road and observe the following safety rules:

- Keep your bike in good repair. Brake levers should fit snugly on the handlebars; seats, handlebars, and wheels should fit tightly in their housings. Replace cracked, peeling, or bulging tires.
- Don't ride on busy streets if you still wobble when you pedal slowly. Ride on the sidewalk (with an eye out for pedestrians) if the street has heavy car traffic. (Note: Riding on the sidewalk is illegal in some cities. This sandwiches you in a conflict between your own safety and the public law.)
- If you ride in the street, ride with the prevailing flow of traffic. Don't ride the wrong way down one-way streets, and don't ride on the wrong side of two-way streets. If there's no bike lane, ride in the right lane, not the parking lane. Don't duck into spaces between parked cars—you'll be invisible to motorists when you pull out again.
- Obey all traffic signals and street signs. Think of yourself as another vehicle on the road.
- Use conventional motorists' hand signals to tell drivers what you plan to do, and then, if possible, make eye contact to make sure they understand—and agree.
- Attach a loud horn to your handlebars or carry a whistle between your teeth. And use it often to make your presence known.
- Don't ride next to a car's right hindquarter. That's the driver's blind spot.
- If you are on a lightly traveled street and you want to turn left or right, move into the appropriate lane, just as if you were a car. If you are riding in a street with heavy traffic, get off your bike at the intersection and cross in the crosswalk as if you were a pedestrian.
- Watch for opening car doors and cars pulling into traffic.
- Watch for potholes, gravel along corner curbs or in the street, soft shoulders, drain grates, cattle guards, and railroad tracks. Avoid riding on wet streets or on wet, soggy, slick, or muddy trails. Beware of wet and slippery lane stripes.
- Don't ride at night—you can't see the potholes, and drivers can't see you. And don't rely too heavily on

reflectorized clothing. Most of it reflects light dimly or only at certain angles. Reflectors on the pedals help a bit. A flashing beacon on your rear rack, flashlights attached to both legs, and a headlight improve your chances, but not enormously.
- If you're riding off-road, stay away from the edges of cliffs and other precipices.

For the Beginner's Cycling Program, see the following page.

# Intermediate Cycling

You are an intermediate cyclist if you ride comfortably three or four times a week for at least an hour each time at a speed of ten to fifteen miles per hour. If all you want is to stay in shape, stay at this level. For variety, join a bike tour of some nearby park or scenic wonder. One of our friends goes cycle birdwatching along the shoreline of San Francisco Bay. "I've always been an ecology buff," Dorothy explains, "but I'm not big on backpacking. Every fall, I bicycle in all the wildlife refuges along the bay. You wouldn't consider any of these rides a workout because every time I see a flock of pelicans or a great blue heron, I stop and stare. Still, I cover a lot of mileage. One ride is about eight miles, another twelve, and so on."

At this level, you're in shape to tour just about anywhere in the world as long as the terrain is fairly flat or dotted with gently rolling hills.

## SPECIAL TIPS

At this point, the following little elements of style make a big difference in your performance:

- Pedal on the ball of your foot instead of the arch or the flat foot. Use lots of ankle motion.
- Move your seat forward or back to increase your efficiency. Ideally, your saddle should be behind the place where the pedals turn around. (A test: If you're sitting on the saddle and one pedal is at its highest and the other at its lowest, a plumb line dropped from your kneecap should fall about three-quarters of an inch behind the pedal.)

## BEGINNER'S CYCLING PROGRAM

| WEEK | MILES | TIME | MILES PER HOUR |
|------|-------|------|----------------|
| 1 | at your ease | at your ease | at your ease |
| 2 | 1 or 2 | at your ease | at your ease |
| 3 | 3 | 18 minutes | 10 |
| 4 | 4 | 24 minutes | 10 |
| 5 | 4 | 20 minutes | 12 |
| 6 | 4 | 18 minutes | 13.5 |
| 7 | 4 | 16 minutes | 15 |
| 8 | 5 | 30 minutes | 10 |
| 9 | 5 | 25 minutes | 12 |
| 10 | 5 | 22 minutes | 13.5 |
| 11 | 5 | 20 minutes | 15 |
| 12 | 6 | 36 minutes | 10 |
| 13 | 6 | 30 minutes | 12 |
| 14 | 6 | 27 minutes | 13.5 |
| 15 | 6 | 24 minutes | 15 |
| 16 | 7 | 42 minutes | 10 |
| 17 | 7 | 35 minutes | 12 |
| 18 | 7 | 31 minutes | 13.5 |
| 19 | 7 | 28 minutes | 15 |
| 20 | 8 | 48 minutes | 10 |
| 21 | 8 | 40 minutes | 12 |
| 22 | 8 | 35 minutes | 13.5 |
| 23 | 8 | 32 minutes | 15 |

Note: On this schedule, you alternate weeks of adding miles with weeks of increasing your speed.

If this moves too quickly, repeat a week as many times as you feel necessary.

After week 23, continue riding eight miles in thirty-two minutes until it feels too easy. Then gradually increase your mileage until you're riding an hour a day, at least three days a week.

- If you own a touring bike with dropped handlebars (ram's horns), your hand position adds or subtracts as much as 14 percent of your efficiency. When you rest your hands on top of the bars, you're only 86 percent as efficient as if you rested them on the drops the way racers do. However, that racer's crouch is death on the back. Compromise by tilting your handlebars so that the drops are angled up a bit—resembling a living ram's horns. This brings the brake levers closer to your hands so you can sit a little more upright.

# Masters Cycling

You are a master cyclist if you can ride three or four days a week for two hours a shot at an eighteen- or nineteen-mile-per-hour pace. By now, you've gone beyond cycling just to stay in shape. If you want to race, ride off-road on mountain trails, or tour the Swiss Alps or the foothills of Mount Everest, you can add hills to your daily rides or do interval training. Either training method improves your power and speed.

For hill training, pick countryside with many small hills so you can ride a short, sharp uphill, then rest on the short, steep downhill. Don't try long, relentless uphill rides until you've been riding short hills for several months.

Interval training on a flat course works on the same principle as short-hill training: you ride as hard as you can for short bursts—say, one minute—then ride slowly until your pulse comes down to your usual huffing-and-puffing level—say another minute—then lay on the steam again. Ride slowly during the rest periods because the incomplete rest builds up your stamina. Work yourself up to ten or fifteen of the hard/easy intervals per workout, but don't do this more than twice a week and never two days in a row. It's an extremely grueling form of training.

There's no point in working much on intervals unless you plan to race in one of the age-graded (formerly called veterans) circuits. After a fifty-year sag, bicycle racing is making a comeback in the United States, although we still have a long way to go to match the fervor of the Europeans, British, and even the Canadians about the sport. Today, throughout the country, you have just about all the racing options you would have had in bicycle racing's heyday in the twenties and thirties:

- *Time trials* in which you race against the clock instead of fellow racers over distances of 10, 25, 30, 50, or 100 miles, or over times of twelve and twenty-four hours.
- *Road racing* either on the road or, less commonly in this country, on specially designed tracks called velodromes. There are various sorts of road races. In massed-start races everyone starts together and the first person across the line is the winner (as in a marathon footrace). When these races are held on a short, flat, circular, or figure-eight course closed off to traffic, they're called criterium races. If they're held on open courses and travel through hilly countryside, they're called open-road races. Another type is the staged race, the most famous of which is the Tour de France. These races cover different types of terrain, include time trials, point-to-point races, and long mountainous climbs. They take place over several days or weeks and sometimes several thousand miles.
- *Track racing* requires a specially designed, very expensive velodrome, such as those in Encino, California; San Jose, California; Portland, Oregon; Shakopee, Minnesota; Kenosha, Wisconsin; Milwaukee, Wisconsin; Northbrook, Illinois; St. Louis, Missouri; and New York, New York. Riders may race in quarter- and half-mile handicap races, 800- and 1,000-meter Olympic-style sprint match-races, 4,000-meter pursuit track races, and several other less popular formats.

To find an organized age-graded cycling program in your area, contact the United States Cycling Federation (see Resources at the back of this book), which sanctions age-graded programs on the local, state, and national levels and is affiliated with the Union Cycliste International, cycling's world governing body, for international races.

## SEEING THE WORLD ON WHEELS

You can see almost the entire world on wheels. Where to begin? Clubs all over the country organize daylong outings or summerlong packaged sightseeing tours across Europe, India, China, and just about any other exotic locale you can name. On most of these tours, you ride about fifty miles a day. A "sagwagon" follows, carrying your luggage and some daytime meals. Lodging each night is in comfortable, first-quality inns and hotels.

Check cycling and nature magazines and travel agents for packages and, if you're over fifty, check the ads in *Modern Maturity* and other retirement magazines. Cycle touring is not just for the young, by any means.

You can, of course, tour on your own. James Wang and two friends spent last summer riding through parts of France and Italy. "Ever since my son toured Europe by bike, I had to try it," Wang says. "We met more people that way than we'd met in all our other trips to Europe combined, and we got to see and smell nature all around us—the farms, the forests, the parks. We rode about eighty miles a day and stayed mostly in little inns. We bought food in markets and delicatessens for lunch but ate in restaurants or sometimes some kind person's house for dinner—and we still lost weight!"

If you're taking your bike abroad, airlines provide bike cartons. Just make sure you bring tools to reassemble your bike at the other end. You can make room reservations every fifty to eighty miles, although many cycle tourists prefer the spontaneity of arriving in a town and looking for lodging. Rarely are you forced to camp out; if there are no rooms, some farmer or policeman will take you in. However, have enough smarts to avoid major holidays and festivals. Unless you like camping out, don't travel in France during August, for example. No one is home and most businesses are closed.

Interested in off-road touring? Tour guides organize back-country tours complete with sagwagon service and, in some cases, hotel lodging instead of camping out. Some even offer mountain bike rentals. Check *Bicycling* magazine and the organization called Bikecentennial (see Resources).

What about cycling on water? A California inventor named Joe Knapp builds canoes modified with low seats and foot-pedaling arrangements similar to a recumbent bicycle. They go like the wind with very little effort and ride along on such an even keel that you can use your hands for whatever important business you have—fishing, say, or eating a picnic lunch. The more loaded with people and gear his boats are (within reason), the more stable they are. Great fun.

# First Aid

**Back pain:** Riding a standard ten-speed bicycle in that bent-over position is hard on the lower back. A ten-dollar elastic lumbosacral belt, available at medical supply stores, supports the abdominal muscles and prevents backaches. Also, get off your bike every thirty minutes and stretch your back muscles. Lie on your back in the grass and pull first one knee, then the other, to your chest.

Other solutions: Readjust your seat higher or lower, move it forward or back, or tilt the nose of it up or down. Or raise or lower your handlebars.

Attempt to avoid back problems entirely by riding upright rather than racer's crouch cycles, be they one- or three-speed bikes, tricycles, or mountain bikes. Also, recumbent bicycles, tricycles, or quadricycles spare your back.

**Sore or numb hands:** If you have arthritis, take two aspirins before you start riding. Keep your hands warm with supple gloves—fingerless, preferably, for best dexterity. Thicken your handlebars and grips with tape or special foam available at bike stores. Wear padded gloves. If you've got a racing-style bike, don't lean too much on the handlebars. Or buy an upright-style bike. Have your brake levers (called calipers) readjusted so you don't have to squeeze as hard. (Don't release them too much or you might get into an accident.) Check your seat-to-handlebar distance. Your elbows should be slightly bent when your hands rest on the middle of your handlebars. If this cramps your neck, have your bike fitted with a larger stem (the tube attaching the handlebars to the bike). Also, be sure that your frame is the right size so you don't have to lean on or grab onto the handlebars too tightly.

**Sore neck:** Check the size of your bike and the distance between the handlebars and the seat. Switch to an upright riding position.

**Sore knees:** Your bicycle is either too big or too small, or your seat is too low. If you have arthritis, strengthen the muscles in the front of your thigh by doing twelve to fifteen repetitions of the following exercise every day:

Sit on a bench or a table. Hang an ankle weight around your instep or dangle it from your pointed toe. If you don't have an ankle weight, try an old purse filled with rocks. Start with a pound weight and move up as the exercise gets easier. Slowly, slowly, straighten your leg so that it's straight from the hip and parallel to the floor.

Slowly, slowly, bend your knee until your lower leg is dangling down. This completes one repetition of the exercise. It's much harder to do this slowly than quickly, but you get a much better workout.

Cycling takes you places. You travel on your bike to far-away places with strange-sounding names—an unfamiliar neighborhood across town or a country lane lined with the red trees of autumn or a Sicilian peasant's farm or a Scottish fishing resort. You forget you're exercising. You're just out enjoying the world from the best seat in the house—a bicycle seat.

# Cross-Country Skiing: Gliding Your Way to Tip-top Condition

**M**ention skiing to most people, and they picture whizzing down mountainsides at terrifying speeds, crashing into trees, and spending the rest of vacation in casts from toes to hips. That's Alpine skiing—fraught with danger and not very aerobic. That's not the kind of skiing we recommend.

We're talking about cross-country skiing, a graceful, gliding kind of sport you do on the snowy flats. The sort of skiing you can get the hang of in five minutes. The sort that takes little skill and no bravery. The safe, aerobic, health-giving skiing. The sport-for-the-whole-family skiing.

"Anyone who can walk and talk at the same time can learn to cross-country ski without a single lesson," says Ellen Dochter. "Let me put it another way: if I can do it, anyone can." A friend taught her to ski right in Ellen's driveway the day after a record snowfall had closed all the streets in Cambridge, Massachusetts. "We just stood next to the garage, and she showed me how to fit my boots into the bindings on the skis, how to use my poles to push myself, and how to slide on one ski, then the other. Then we skied down one of Cambridge's main streets. It was like time had stopped. It was supernatural."

# The Pitch

Cross-country (or Nordic) skiing is simply an elegant—and inexpensive—way of hiking across flat, snowy plains, whether they are high meadows in the Sierra or isolated country roads in Vermont. With skis, you follow the snow along hiking and biking trails, bridle paths, up and down the fairways of the local golf course. The boots and skinny cross-country skis are so comfortable, they don't seem to require any sort of balance. Because the skis hinge to the boot only at the toe, your foot moves freely and naturally, almost as if you're walking. You slide smoothly and gently on top of the snow. Five minutes of experimenting and you've got the idea. Then, of course, you'll spend a lifetime perfecting your style. No expensive admission passes, no long lines, no ski lifts, and no expensive and intimidating equipment.

Nordic skiing is a great workout, but that's not why people ski. They ski because it's so easy to learn and it's so much fun. And they love the fact that they can ski with their entire families, side by side, mile after mile, hour after hour—grandmother, mother, father, teenagers, and younger children together. How many Alpine skiing families can do that?

Cross-country skiing is taking off. New resorts are popping up all over, and established resorts say their business has doubled or tripled in the last three years. Nordic touring centers and other resorts and national parks with prepared ski tracks are the easiest places to learn. The tracks themselves are very smooth, machine-cut grooves, and most resorts have separate trails for beginners and advanced skiers. In addition, most winter recreation centers have beginner's classes.

Still, to us, the best part of cross-country skiing is literally skiing across country. We like to set out on our own across some nice flat field or down some country lane. There's a special thrill to following fox tracks down a logging road or coming upon a rabbit beside a frozen pond. We've met deer. We've met an ice fisherman (who thought *we* were nuts).

We've met a large family cutting their Christmas trees. Only rarely have we met other skiers.

You can find a rare sort of peace while skiing, along with an incredible exhilaration. Every part of your body, but especially your heart and lungs, gets a superior workout. Cross-country skiing is probably the most aerobic sport of all, yet you feel no strain. Your movements flow outward, softly and easily, drawing on the bones and muscles, with none of the impact, up-and-down pounding, or wrenching effort you often experience during hard-surface activities. Yet every muscle tingles, every part of your body is tightened and toned. You get long, sleek, durable arm, shoulder, back, chest, abdominal, hip, buttocks, thigh, and lower leg muscles. Injuries are rare and usually happen when skiers try to ski down hills before they're ready. In fact, exercise physiologists say that cross-country skiing is the best all-around workout there is.

Because skiing is smooth, not jarring, most people with back trouble and arthritis can ski Nordic comfortably. In fact, Ron has a friend with such severe rheumatoid arthritis that he has great difficulty walking, yet he skis easily and relatively painlessly. Cross-country skiing is good aerobic exercise for people with heart conditions. However, you must start out slowly because you are using your arms as well as your legs, and any arm exercise spikes up your heart rate. It's even good for those of you with asthma or other lung conditions, as long as you take sensible precautions to prevent an attack. Wear a mouthless ski mask to warm and moisturize the air you breathe, and ask your doctor about inhalants to use just before you start skiing.

**Don't cross-country ski without a doctor's approval if** you have Ménière's disease, which impairs your sense of balance.

# Buying and Testing Your Equipment

In order to cross-country ski, you need poles with wrist straps, skis, and comfortable Nordic ski boots (they look a lot like hiking boots, but their toes fasten onto metal hinges on the skis). Cross-country ski equipment is inexpensive to rent or to buy. For occasional skiing, we recommend renting from any reputable local sporting goods or ski shop. If you rent skis more than five times a winter, however, you might as well buy, because the rental fees will add up to the cost of a complete, moderately priced skiing package. A moderately priced package should run between $150 and $300 to buy and $7 a day to rent.

If you decide to purchase equipment, here are a few things to look for. Most skis nowadays are made of fiberglass laid over a core of wood, foam, or plastic. (Wooden skis, like wooden boats, are beautiful but very expensive.) You'll have to choose between waxless or waxable skis. Until a few years ago, all skis had to be waxed or they would slip and skid instead of track and slide. Today, you'll find a wide choice of waxless skis, but none of them is perfect. Although they're the height of convenience—you just put them on and go—and they glide fairly well over most kinds of snow, they don't work perfectly on any. They tend to accumulate thick, sticky layers of snow on their bottoms and slip miserably on even the smallest hills. Waxless skis are a boon if you're skiing in the West, where snow conditions change every quarter mile or so, but they aren't as useful where temperature and snow conditions are fairly predictable and waxing once in the morning gets you through the whole day.

If you choose waxable skis, you'll find waxing surprisingly simple. Waxes are color-coded. Just choose the appropriate one for the outdoor temperature and then crayon it lightly on the bottoms of both skis, an exercise of perhaps forty seconds. Rub the wax in with the side of a cork block or an old wine cork, and that's all there is to it. If you notice you slip on the snow, or that you don't slide at all but get stuck in mid-glide, figure you've worn off your wax or used the wrong one. Pull the wax out of your pocket and redo it.

Beyond choosing between waxless and waxable skis, the technical aspects of ski construction become arcane. If you're just renting for a couple of days, tell the salesperson what kind of skiing you're going to do, track skiing or off-track touring, and take whatever package the store provides.

If you're buying, opt for skis that will work for both track and off-track skiing unless you're certain you'll do only one type. To determine how long your skis should be, stand with one arm up in the air. The tip of your ski should just touch your wrist. Touring skis are arched in the center. Get a ski with enough springiness to flatten the arch out when you put all

your weight on one ski, but not so soft that it flattens when you
stand with your weight evenly distributed on both skis. Should
someone try to sell you skis with metal edges, walk away. Metal
edges are only for downhill cross-country skiing, and that's way
beyond all of us.

Your boots must be more comfortable than running shoes.
Look for nice broad toe boxes with room for your toes to
wriggle, and for flexible soles that bend the way walking shoes
do. Boots should be waterproof, should have collars around the
ankle and instep to block the snow, and should provide padding and support around the ankle. We also recommend wearing insulated innersoles to keep your feet warm. (Bring them
along when you try on your boots.)

Each brand of boot is designed to work with a particular
binding system. That means you have to buy the correct bindings to fit your boots. For recreational skiing, the toe or "rat
trap" style of binding is best. Two or three holes in the toe of
your boot fit into two or three pins in the binding, and then the
boot toe is held in place with a wire contraption. The binding,
in turn, is anchored to the ski. This binding permits you the
freest of strides, because you can lift practically the whole boot
except the very toe off the ski.

After boots and bindings, all you need are a couple of
poles. Pick whatever pole, grip, and strap combination feels
good, be it fiberglass, metal, or fiberglass/graphite. Buy adjustable straps, because you may wear varying thicknesses of
gloves or mittens, depending on the weather. The pole should
reach about two inches below the top of your shoulders.

Nordic ski machines give you an extraordinary workout in
the warmth of your living room. See Chapter 9 for details.

# Clothing

You need no special ski clothes. Just be sure to dress in layers:
you'll want to peel down once you've worked up a sweat, but
you may also need to pile on the down if the weather turns
chilly. The traditional Nordic ski outfit starts with some sort of
wickable thermal underwear. The outer layers consist of
knickers, heavy knee socks, turtleneck wool sweater over a
cotton shirt, and a ski cap with a pompom—and ear flaps if
possible. However, some prefer the slick body suit Nordic

outfits, and others wear any old pair of blue jeans. Whatever works.

We recommend waterproof gaiters to keep your legs and feet dry. These look like baggy outer leggings and run from the knee to the top of the laces of the boot. Also wear two pairs of socks—similar in thickness to the two pairs you wore when you tried on your boots. The inner pair not only keeps your feet warm but also wicks away perspiration. Unless you plan to ski in bad weather, a dumb move unless you're a trained survivalist, you probably won't need a waterproof shell. But you may wish to carry a lightweight windproof shell and a scarf to cover your nose and mouth in case an icy wind comes up (see Chapter 3).

You'll need good, tough, warm gloves. However, don't buy stiff ones. The effort of bending the gloves as you grip the poles gives you terrible hand cramps after a while. Tight gloves will cut off the circulation in your clenched fists, chilling your hands and leaving them numb.

Always wear sunglasses and sunscreen. The snow reflects ultraviolet and infrared rays as much or more than the water and sand at the beach (see Chapter 4).

# Warming Up

Warm up your heart with five to ten minutes of easy skiing and only a little poling. (Too much arm effort will spike your heart rate too high too soon.) Cool off the same way at the end of your skiing day. If you're stiff four hours or more after skiing, stretch before and after skiing from then on.

It may be cold outside, but you're going to work up a sweat. Drink lots of water before you set out and drink water again when you get home. If you plan to ski for more than an hour, carry a thermos in a backpack and stop frequently for a drink of something hot or cold (see Chapter 4).

# The Basics

Just put on your skis and go. You'll spend the first day getting the hang of gliding and poling, but after an hour or so, you'll be sailing along, unaware of how far you've gone.

## FIVE-MINUTE LESSON

With these instructions, you'll be off and skiing on your first day. For the finer points, the techniques you'll need as an intermediate or masters skier, ask an expert skier friend or take lessons at a Nordic center.

To get the feel of the skis, start out walking on them. You'll find this very discouraging. Walking is much harder work than skiing, because it takes a lot of effort to lift a ski almost off the ground and take a step. Use your poles for balance if necessary. Don't spend too much time on this first step because you want to get on with the fun stuff.

Now try this. Think of your right ski as a scooter. Shift most of your weight onto your left foot and push down and backward with your left ski. Your right ski will glide forward a bit. Now, shift your weight to your right foot, press down on your right ski and slide on your left. Right, left, right . . . (In confusing Nordic skiing parlance, the pressing-down part of this motion is called the kick. The gliding part, more logically, is called the glide.) This motion feels like ice skating, or even roller skating, but your heel comes up off the ski as your foot moves behind you. Use your poles for balance.

It's not all that easy. It takes courage to shift your weight almost entirely onto one ski and then almost entirely onto the other. Practice that a while until you move more freely.

Now, start using your poles to move you along. If you let your poles do at least 10 percent of the work, you'll be able to ski a lot farther before you get tired. You want to use your right pole to pull the future toward you while you use your right ski to glide into it. (Think of the scooter again. When you were a kid, did you ever sit on a scooter and scoot it along with your hands instead of your feet? You reached ahead with your hands and pushed the ground back in order to roll the scooter forward. That's what you're doing with your ski poles.) Lean forward a bit from the waist (only as far as is comfortable), bend your knees a little, and plant your pole beside your ski and twelve inches or so ahead of your body. The poles move almost in circles parallel to your body, as if you were a car and they were two giant wheels rolling you forward. Don't stick the poles out to the sides. As you glide forward on the ski, thrust backward with the pole. Some say it feels as if you are using your arms to swim through the snow. Others say the poles feel like propellers.

That's all there is to it. As you get better, you'll master techniques to make you more efficient, you'll lean out farther with your poles, your arms and legs will work fluidly together, and your glides will get longer.

Lean your body at a forty-five-degree angle and keep your head up and your eyes focused ten or fifteen feet ahead of you. Watching the road not only keeps you from crashing into trees and rocks but also keeps you from arching too far forward.

Keep your knees slightly bent, just enough to keep you stable with your weight over the center of the ski. Put your weight a little more onto the ball than the heel of your foot. This bends your ankle forward and centers your weight. (If you let your weight settle onto your heels, you won't be able to glide, but you will be able to fall.)

Swing your arms naturally, the way you do when you walk: as your left ski moves forward, your right arm moves forward. Keep your arm bent during the forward part of your poling stroke. Don't reach forward so far that you have to straighten your arm completely. When you push off with your pole, put some shoulder in it to give it extra oomph. Once you've pushed off, let go of the pole. Don't worry: the strap around your wrist will keep it in place. If your straps are adjusted correctly, the handle will stay between your thumb and forefinger. When you let go of the pole, your arm is free to move forward naturally. If you keep a tight grip on it, you don't reach out as far. As you let go of the pole, let your arm continue its backward swing until it's almost straight before you bring it forward again. This is the same motion you use when you walk.

The biggest problem of cross-country skiing, after finding snow, is getting good enough at skiing before the season ends. Preseason training on dry land during the fall will help you make greater strides, as it were, during the winter.

To ski-walk, find some hills. (Don't try this unless you're in good enough shape to walk up hills briskly.) Stride up them imitating your skiing motion. Take long strides, bending your leading leg at the knee and keeping your trailing leg as straight as possible. Transfer your weight fully from one leg to the next. Push down against the ground, not back against the hill. (If you pushed back on skis, you'd slide backward down the hill.) Use your arms as if you were poling. Bring, say, your right arm forward as you stride out with your left leg; then bring your left arm forward with your right leg. This is called working in opposition. Keep your arms slightly bent and bring your hand up to eye level each time, as if you were holding a ski pole. If you are lucky enough to find some unpaved hills, use actual ski poles, the way you would in skiing, to help pull your weight up the hill.

Speaking of hills, try to avoid them as a beginner. If you have no choice, don't try to ski down them. Take off your skis and walk down unless you are a skilled Alpine (or downhill) skier. Otherwise, you're likely to break some part of your body. Uphills aren't as treacherous, but they're hard work on skis. You have to duck-walk up them, pointing each ski outward at a forty-five-degree angle and cutting into the snow with the inside edges, all the while pulling yourself up with your poles. This is called herringboning.

## SCHEDULE

Stop to rest frequently. You'll work up a sweat and get your heart pumping from the combination of arm and leg exertion. (Don't overuse your arms or you'll poop out almost immediately.) As you get better, you'll ski for longer and longer periods and take fewer and shorter breaks.

At first, stay near your car or some other home port. As you become more confident, venture farther, but remember, you've got to ski as many miles home as you skied out.

As an aerobic workout, cross-country skiing is a special case. On the one hand, it is one of the two most complete aerobic and toning exercises on earth. (Rowing is the other.) On the other hand, very few people see enough snow to cross-country ski every other day, week after week, for four or six months a year. Except for those few, even the most obsessive skier skis only on weekends. For this reason, you can't maintain a training program for cross-country skiing the way you can for the other sports in Part Three. Your goal, therefore, is to become a good enough skier to have fun with it whenever you get the chance, and get a model workout at the same time.

If you're skiing for the exercise, aim at being able to ski thirty to sixty minutes nonstop. However, once you're in good shape, you're not going to want to quit after an hour. What's the point of going to all that trouble, renting skis, schlepping them to the snow, getting yourself all kitted out, just to ski for a few minutes? If you ski only occasionally, don't attempt a daylong excursion unless you're certain you're in good shape.

Instead, take two shorter ski trips, one in the morning and another after lunch.

# Intermediate Skiing

Consider yourself an intermediate skier if you've mastered the kick and glide step, also known as the diagonal stride (a confusing name if we ever heard one, considering that your skis stay parallel as you move forward). With well-coordinated poling, you move smoothly and effortlessly, sliding along the snow like a graceful tractor.

Now is the time to take lessons at a Nordic ski center or from an outdoor or environmental group. You should learn how to herringbone up hills (so you don't slide backward) and snowplow and half-wedge your way down (so you stay in control).

From now on, you are probably strong enough to take on modest all-day trips—just you, your friends, and a backpack full of hot coffee and substantial sandwiches. Start with seven- or eight-milers (round-trip), with almost no hills. As that gets easier, work yourself up to ten or twelve miles with only moderate elevation changes—say, a total of 800 feet, up and down, for the whole trip. Remember, the difficulty of a trip depends not just on the distance but on the steepness of the hills you climb and ski down. Buy a local guidebook from an outdoors equipment store, or buy a topographic map and make sure you understand it. Now you're also in good enough shape to join one of the day excursions organized by ski touring companies or the Sierra Club.

# Masters Skiing

You are a master skier if, in addition, you use the short, crisp, diagonal uphill stride to actually ski up hills instead of herringboning them and if you can snowplow or half-wedge yourself down hills with complete control. Now is the time to take lessons to learn Telemark and Christie turns, two maneuvers that take great skill but, once mastered, make downhill and convoluted trail skiing much easier.

By the time you get to this level, you'll probably have heard a lot about skating, a track-racing technique that's all the rage. Both types of skating—marathon and V-skating—require terrific conditioning, great balance, and wonderful rhythm. When you marathon skate, you keep one ski in the track while you angle the other outward and drive its inner edge into the snow to push you forward. When you V-skate, both skis are angled outward, much like the herringbone. Skating is about 20 percent faster than striding—important if you're racing, not so important otherwise. If you plan to skate, don't wax your skis for good grip on the snow. You don't want any grip at all—it slows you down. And don't try it on anything but hard-packed snow. It just doesn't work on anything else.

You might enjoy participating in a citizen's race, so-called because the entrants are recreational rather than racing skiers. These are scheduled throughout the country under auspices of the U.S. Ski Association.

If you're a master skier, you may be tempted to strike out on your own, blazing a trail through magnificent and unspoiled wilderness. Fine. You're probably in shape for it. Just make sure you know how to read a topographic map, use a compass, and survive overnight in icy temperatures if you get lost. If you're not an expert at all three, don't go by yourself. Join an organized group tour or hire a professional and well-recommended private guide.

## SEEING THE WORLD ON SKINNY SKIS

The Sierra Club, many vacation tour groups, many local ski clubs, and many ski resorts offer organized day and weekend ski tours in most of our snowy states—Alaska, the Sierra and Rockies states, New England, Michigan, even Hawaii (yes, Hawaii—on volcanoes of the Big Island). Similar trips are available in Canada, the Scandinavian countries, parts of Japan, and in South America—a chance to ski in summer, which is winter there. Contact the Ski Touring Council, the U.S. Ski Association, or read the ads and articles in *Cross Country Skier* (see Resources). Or ask a nearby ski outfitter or resort for the names and phone numbers of local ski clubs. Some clubs are quite specific—restricted to singles, or couples over fifty, or tourers (no racers).

# First Aid

**Cold injury:** Frostbite is one problem that, barring unforeseen circumstances, is preventable. Just stay away from tracked or untracked wilderness when the wind-chill factor drops below zero. Conversely, if you don't dress warmly enough, or if you're caught in a sudden storm, or if your clothes are wet from sweat or melting snow, you may suffer hypothermia. See the Taking the Chill Out of Cold Weather section in Chapter 4 for complete information on frostbite and hypothermia.

**Sore knees:** See the First Aid section in Chapter 15.

**Arthritic pain in hands from gripping the poles:** Wrap foam around the grips to thicken them. Wear silk glove liners under your mittens for extra insulation. Take a couple of aspirin before skiing.

**Osteoporosis:** If you have this condition—and many people over fifty-five do to some degree—learn how to fall. Fall back on your rear rather than forward or sideways. Don't put out your hand to catch your fall unless you want a fractured wrist.

Cross-country skiing has it all over Alpine skiing. Cross-country is a snap to learn. It's safe. It's marvelously aerobic. If you want solitude, you can ski happily by yourself—no crowds, no ski lifts, no hassles. If you want company, the whole family can go along and everyone will be able to keep up. And, best of all, when you Nordic ski, you feel as if you're part of the woods and meadows, as if you're barely disturbing the life around you. That's a package that's hard to beat.

# CHAPTER 17

# Rowing, Canoeing, and Kayaking: Nature's Complete, Total, and Perfect Exercise

It's a shame more people don't know how easy and exhilarating rowing, canoeing, and kayaking are. Not only are they missing out on a stunning feeling of personal satisfaction and pride, but they're also missing out on some extraordinary health benefits.

When we first hear about paddling around on the water, we figure it takes too much courage or some sort of special skill. Not true at all. If it were so difficult, it wouldn't be nearly as popular. And popular it is. If you don't believe us, drive along the highway toward a family resort one Friday and count the number of dinghies and canoes strapped to the tops of the trailers and RVs.

You don't need special skills or expensive classes. Rowing a boat or paddling a canoe or kayak takes only a few minutes to learn from an experienced friend or instructor and only a little longer to learn from our Five-Minute Lesson. And once you try it, you'll be hooked for a lifetime.

# The Pitch for Rowing

Are you among the millions who, at some time in your youth, tried to row an old wooden bathtub across a lake and succeeded only in sending the boat round and round in a tight little circle? If so, you probably are about to turn the page. You don't need that kind of humiliation again, not at your age, right?

Forget the bad old days. You don't have to be Arnold Schwarzenegger to be able to glide across a quiet bay, watch the blue herons in the sky above you, and feel the excitement and tranquility of one of nature's few complete, total, and perfect exercises. In one of today's lightweight rowing shells with a sliding seat, you use your strong legs to *push* the boat through the water while your arms *pull* the oars. Your whole body propels you through the water, and that makes the work a lot easier.

It's true that rowing requires skill, but it's skill that's easily learned. About 70 percent of rowing comes from logical body movement. You get the hang of it quickly, but the thrill lasts a lifetime.

Rowing requires discipline and dedication but rewards you with continual growth. You get better and better the longer you row. It is harder work than running or walking, but more addictive. Once you've rowed for a few months, not to mention a few years, you won't be able to give it up.

"I've never found anything that feeds all the senses the way rowing does," says Mike Peabody, a fifty-six-year-old stock analyst. "You smell the water. You taste the air. You hear the heartbeatlike rhythm of your oars. You feel the boat part the water. And you see everything.

"I've been rowing on and off—mostly on—since college days," he says, "and it has meant different things to me at different times in my life. When I was younger, I thrived on the competition. Now, I like the solitude. I can't think of anything more exhilarating than cutting across a quiet bay, just me and the cormorants and the seals.

"I stopped rowing for a few years after college. When I came back to it, crew had lost its appeal for me. Now, I just want to row for myself. I know there are masters races for older crews, but I don't know many people who get into that.

I just want to be out on the water. It's so calm and quiet and different from my office and my everyday life. The quieter it is, the better I like it."

Rowing is supremely aerobic. In fact, it's right up there at the top of aerobic exercises, second only to cross-country skiing. It strengthens your heart and lungs, burns more calories, expends more energy, improves oxygen uptake quicker, speeds up your metabolism more effectively.

For example, rowing one mile provides about the same aerobic benefits as running a mile and a quarter because you use most of your major muscle groups when you row instead of just the few leg muscles used in running. Rowing limbers and firms up your entire body—tightening your buttocks, back, abdomen, the fronts of your thighs (called the quadriceps muscles), and most of your upper body. Not even swimming uses as many muscle groups.

Rowing brings another bonus: The muscles you build by rowing are long and lean. Even the burliest male college crew members look lean compared to swimmers or football players. And the legs of women who go out for crew in high school and college are long, firm, and shapely. (Runners' legs, by contrast, tend to get ropy, while bicyclists develop huge, bulky thighs with bulges just above the knee.)

Rowing firms and tightens so smoothly because there's no strain to the muscles or joints—you sit down while the water yields to your oars and the boat slides along. Your movements are horizontal, gliding, and smooth so you don't pull and tear parts of your body. No impact, no jolts, no jarring, no huge forces pounding at your feet and legs as in running and even, to a lesser extent, walking. The rhythmic, regular movements of your oar strokes alternately relax and contract your muscles. This promotes even circulation, pumps away tissue wastes more efficiently, and is ultimately more tranquilizing than jarring, jerky motions. Many people who can't stand, walk, or run can sit and row. This makes it highly suitable for people with arthritis, stress incontinence, and some circulatory problems (with doctor's permission, of course). What's more, doctors now recommend rowing to cardiac patients and people with low back and disk problems. (The back question is tricky. Rowing helps some back problems but aggravates others. Ask your doctor.)

Rowing, like cycling, offers the fascination of working with finely crafted equipment. Whether you rent or buy, you may feel obligated by the financial outlay to keep at it. But that's not all. Water has a primitive attraction. It's always different, changing currents, colors, plant and animal life. There's always something new to learn. That's why so many rowers are in their seventies or eighties and a few are even in their nineties —they've been rowing most of their lives and still have more to learn.

Almost every town has some rowable body of water—a quiet river bathed in morning mists, a lagoon in a city park, a bay, or an inlet. If you can't find rowable water near you, call a local rowing club. Sometimes they're listed in the white pages of the telephone book as Your Town's Rowing Club or Your Town's Athletic Club or Your Town's Swimming and Rowing Club. Or look in the Yellow Pages under Boats, Renting and Leasing; Boats, Dealers; or Boating Instruction. Someone at one of these businesses can give you the number of the local rowing club or Sierra Club. Or write to the United States Rowing Association (see Resources at the back of this book) for a list of member clubs.

Rowing clubs and other outdoors groups offer weekend day trips and picnics. They provide lessons, as well as companionship, and a chance to make new friends while you exercise. Boating clubs also provide safety in numbers. It's dangerous to go out in a boat by yourself. If you capsize alone, no one will know for hours.

Admittedly, there are minuses. Rowing is too complicated an operation to take up just for your health. ("You don't row because it's good for you," says Eleanor Peabody, Mike's wife, "any more than you bake homemade bread because it's good for you. You row because you love it.") First of all, you've got to rent or buy a proper boat. You've got to find a place to store it, and, if that storage isn't near the water, you've got to haul your boat to and from the water. Worst of all—unless you're an absolute fanatic—rain, wind, and cold will keep you out of your boat for days or months. Still, those bright, crisp days on the water make it all worthwhile.

**Don't row without a doctor's approval if** you have severe back problems, such as advanced degenerative disk disease or spinal arthritis.

# Buying and Testing Your Rowing Equipment

Try rowing an old-fashioned rowboat and you'll know why they're called bathtubs. Your arms, shoulders, and back do all the work, pulling the oars at such odd angles that your back aches after only a few strokes and your arms give out three feet from shore.

What we're talking about here is a recreational rowing shell, a sculling boat: a narrow, maneuverable boat with a seat that slides back and forth on rails or tracks so you can use your legs as well as your arms. You've got a choice of single, double, and four-person boats, but we recommend the single. You don't want to have to scrounge up a partner every time you want to go out on the water. Nevertheless, rowing doubles is a rare experience. It gives you an extraordinary sense of companionship and teamwork.

The classic *racing shells* look like needles floating on the water. They are long (about eighteen feet for a single; twenty-four feet for a double) and narrow and ride fairly high. They're "tippy" because they don't have a keel. Unless you're an old pro, look for the less expensive, wider, more stable and maneuverable *recreational shell.* And, if you're looking for the ultimate unsinkable, untippable boat, it's hard to beat the *rowing catamarans.* They look like great big Hs: two unsinkable pontoons form the verticals of the H, and a canvas sling and sliding seat arrangement make up the H's crossbar. (You sit on the crossbar.)

At this writing, a fiberglass recreational single shell will cost upwards of $1,500; top-of-the-line singles cost about $3,500 to $4,000, and wooden versions hover in the $4,000 range. Obviously, the best plan is to rent from public or private rowing clubs or dealers until you know whether you want to commit to such a purchase.

A rowing machine provides an extraordinary full-body workout and builds strength and aerobic endurance. Use it to supplement your outdoor rowing or as a training regimen unto itself. See Chapter 8.

# Clothing for Rowing

Wear any kind of clothes and shoes you wish, as long as they don't rub against your skin or chafe. And don't forget the hat and sunglasses. Keep them on your head and out of the water with a headband or neckstrap, and attach a bobber to the frames or strap just in case they do fall in. If the weather is even moderately cool, dress in layers, preferably with a waterproof outer shell, because you'll create your own wind-chill factor as you row (see Chapter 4).

Whether or not you know how to swim, wear a Coast Guard rated life jacket (personal flotation device) when you row. The Coast Guard categorizes life jackets into the following five types, rated according to buoyancy:

*Type I:* the most buoyant. They will turn most unconscious people in the water from a face-down position to an upright position and keep victims floating slightly on their backs with their faces well out of the water. They are best to use if you will be far away from the shore or other boats and so may have to float for a long time before rescue. They come in two sizes, adult (more than ninety pounds) and child (less than ninety pounds), and are unwieldy to wear when exercising.

*Type II:* a little less buoyant and will not turn very heavy, unconscious people. They will hold the victim in the same position as Type I. They are best used in areas where rescue is likely to be quick. They come in several sizes and are a little more comfortable.

*Type III:* less buoyant yet, but generally safe for conscious people to use. In this jacket, wearers can place themselves in the ideal vertical and tilted-back position, and the jacket will help them maintain this posture. They are the most comfortable because they allow your arms to move freely without chafing. The Coast Guard notes that Type IIIs are "usually the best choice for water sports, such as skiing, hunting, fishing, canoeing, and kayaking." They come in several sizes according to chest and weight range and are acceptable for use in areas where rescue is likely to be quick.

*Types IV and V* are not safe enough to use.

# Warming Up for Rowing

Rowing may be one of the few sports that require you to stretch. Because you have to reach and bend and then apply a force to your muscles, you may feel a strain or get stiff if you don't do the No-Stress Super Stretches (Chapter 3) before you get into your boat. Whether you need to stretch depends on your build. If rowing without stretching feels uncomfortable or if you're sore the next day, stretch before your aerobic warm-up and after your cool-down.

Once out on the water, paddle around easily for three to five minutes to warm up your heart. When you're done rowing for the day, cool down with the same lazy paddling for another five to ten minutes. When you return to dry land, stretch again with the No-Stress Super Stretches, if you need them.

# The Basics of Rowing

### FIVE-MINUTE LESSON

If you can find a place to take rowing lessons, you're miles ahead at the start. Most rowing teachers provide wide, stable, semi-tubby learning rowboats and show you in a few minutes techniques that take pages to describe. If you can't find a teacher, don't despair. Many rowers insist that anyone can teach himself to row. It will just take longer to get the hang of it.

Practice on a calm, flat, completely predictable stretch of water free from currents. Even modestly turbulent water is dangerous unless you're a strong rower and have experience reading the water.

To get into your boat, sit on the dock, swing your feet onto the footbrace, put one hand on the slide track, and swing your rear end into the seat. Try to keep your weight over the center of the boat. (Unless you know you can step on the floorboards of your boat, don't. It's possible to put your foot all the way through.)

Adjust the footbrace so that the seat stops an inch or two before it hits the blocks at the ends of the rails. Hold the oars so that the inside of the cupped surface faces up. You balance the boat by pressing an oar blade against the water. That lifts up the left side of the boat.

**The stroke.** Practice your first few strokes without using the sliding seat.

1. Grab your oar handles. They overlap. Keep the left (port) handle above the right (starboard) handle.
2. Turn the handles so that the oar blades are flat and parallel to the water. Keep your legs straight so the seat can't move.
3. Bend at the waist and straighten your arms. The oar blades will move behind you toward the front (bow) of the boat.
4. Rotate the handles so that the blades are perpendicular to the water and just above the surface. Raise the oar handles so the blades dip just far enough below the surface to be covered by the water. Don't go any deeper.
5. Pull. The beginning of the pull is called "hitting the catch."
6. As you start to pull, bend your arms, and start to lean back and straighten your back simultaneously. Keep pulling with your arms, leaning and straightening your back until you're about fifteen degrees past upright. Ideally, you should reach the point just as your hands touch your chest. (If this hurts your back, lean back only until you're upright and vertical.) Through all of this, try to keep your wrists straight. That's the end of one stroke. Pause a moment while the boat glides forward.

    Amazing! The boat is moving! Now you've got to get the oars back to the beginning so you can start another stroke. The idea is to move the oars out of the water and through the air without getting them caught in water or wind.
7. To this end, rotate your wrists (which are still up at your chest) to turn the backs of your hands toward your face and the palms toward the back (stern) of the boat. At the same time, push your hands away from your chest and down toward your knees. All of this pulls the oar blades out of the water and turns them flat so they skim the water. This is called "feathering" the oars. The blades are flat the way they were

when you started, and you can use them again, if
necessary, to balance yourself, just as you did in the
beginning.

8. As you push your hands down and away, lean forward again, bend your back, straighten your arms,
and skim the oar blade along the surface of the water.
Don't let it dig into the water. That can slow you
down and even tip you over. Don't let the blade turn
vertical, or it becomes a kite to be blown about by the
wind.

You're ready to hit the catch again. Repeat this stroke
slowly and carefully until you get good enough so that (1) both
oars enter and leave the water at the same moment and (2)
every stroke is even and rhythmic. When you get it right, the
boat will shoot forward, evenly balanced and straight as an
arrow. You want to stroke so rhythmically that the boat never
seems to buck, jerk, plow, or stop. It just coasts ever forward.

One small hint that will make a giant difference in your
balance: Always keep your head up and your eyes forward.
(Actually, they're backward, looking at where you've been, not
where you're going, but let's not get bogged down with details.) Even the wrong angle of your head can affect your balance.

**Leg work.** When you're comfortable with the stroke, add
the legs to get more power with much less effort. At step 3,
bring your legs up against your body until your shins are nearly
vertical and your knees are pressed against your chest between your arms.

At step 5, begin by straightening your legs instead of bending your arms. Leave your arms straight. This way, the power
of this part of the stroke comes from your legs. Let the seat
slide back. When your legs straighten enough so your hands
are over your knees, start leaning back.

When your legs are just about straight, pull in with your
arms as in step 6.

Your hands should arrive at your chest at the same moment your legs straighten fully and the seat reaches the limit
of its slide. (Don't lock your knees or you may hurt them.) The
arm drive and leg drive should start at the same time and stop
at the same time. If your leg drive ends first, it's called "shoot-
ing the slide," and it slows down the movement of the boat.
(Remember to stop your lean when you're about fifteen de-

grees past the vertical unless it hurts your back. If it hurts, lean back only until you're upright and vertical.) And through all of this, try to keep your wrists straight.

That's the end of one stroke. Pause to let the boat glide forward.

In step 7, to get the oars back to the beginning for another stroke and to get your legs bent up under your armpits again, curve your back slightly as your hands pass your knees, lean forward, and slide the seat smoothly forward so that your knees bend toward your chest. Keep the oar blades flat and just skimming the water.

Stop the slide when your shins are vertical and your knees are pressed up against your chest. Now you're ready for the next stroke.

Add power at the beginning of each stroke—when you hit the catch—by punching with your legs, arms, and shoulders. Taper off toward the end of the stroke so the release is clean and you don't have to fight the blade out of the water.

During the release and recovery toward the catch, you shouldn't feel as if you're doing any work. The boat should feel as if it is running out the slide all by itself.

As you practice, try to row the same number of strokes every minute but increase the distance you glide between strokes.

## SCHEDULE

It's going to take you a couple of hours, spread over one to four sessions, to coordinate hitting the catch, feathering the oars, sliding the seat, and balancing the boat. During this first stage, you'll be moving very slowly, so you're not going to get much of an aerobic workout. Don't worry about it. You'll progress quickly.

It's easy to overexert yourself when rowing. Start out slowly. Put in only enough effort to move you across the water and warm you up. Keep your rowing at the gently huffing-and-puffing level. If you feel the need to stop and rest, ship your oars and float for a minute or two. After a while, you'll be rowing farther and faster, enjoying it more, and resting less.

Try to get yourself to the point where you can row about a mile in about half an hour nonstop. You probably won't want to stop at thirty minutes, and that's fine. Row for as long as you like, but remember to leave yourself enough energy to get back to shore.

## BOATING SAFETY TIPS

Most boating accidents happen to novices who never bothered to learn these commonsense rules for living safely on the water.

- Always wear a Coast Guard rated life jacket.
- Always row on calm, flat, predictable water, free from currents. The slightest wave or crosscurrent may capsize your boat.
- Always row or paddle parallel to shore (not straight out to sea) and close enough so that someone will see you if you capsize.
- Never go boating alone. If you violate this cardinal rule, at least, as a poor second, make sure someone knows where you're boating, when you left for the water, and when you plan to be back.
- If your boat turns over, stay with it. Don't try to swim to shore. Your boat is likely to be much more visible than you are. Also, you may swim so far afield that no one will be able to find you.
- Learn how to rescue others. If you don't know safe and effective rescue techniques, you as rescuer may go down with the rescuee—an extremely common occurrence.
- Learn to read the water to avoid rocks, shallows, and treacherous currents.
- Watch the skies and get to shore before a squall comes up. Don't try to beat it or ride it out.
- If a wind comes up before you reach shore, turn your bow into it. Don't let the wind hit you broadside or it will toss you about like a twig.
- When a wave or wake from another boat approaches, turn your bow into it so that your boat is perpendicular to the wave. If it hits you broadside, it will capsize your boat.

## BEGINNER'S ROWING PROGRAM

| WEEK | ROW (IN MINUTES) | REST (IN MINUTES) | REPEATS | TOTAL ROWING TIME |
|---|---|---|---|---|
| 1* | at your leisure | at your leisure | | |
| 2 | at your leisure | at your leisure | | |
| 3 | 3 | 2** | 6 | 18 |
| 4 | 4 | 2 | 5 | 20 |
| 5 | 4 | 1 | 5 | 20 |
| 6 | 5 | 2 | 4 | 20 |
| 7 | 5 | 1 | 4 | 20 |
| 8 | 6 5 | 2 | 3 | 23 |
| 9 | 6 | 1 | 4 | 24 |
| 10 | 7 6 | 2 | 3 | 27 |
| 11 | 7 6 | 1 | 3 | 27 |
| 12 | 8 6 | 2 | 3 | 30 |
| 13 | 8 6 | 1 | 3 | 30 |
| 14 | 9 3 | 2 | 3 | 30 |
| 15 | 9 3 | 1 | 3 | 30 |
| 16 | 10 | 2 | 3 | 30 |
| 17 | 10 | 1 | 3 | 30 |
| 18 | 15 | 3 | 2 | 30 |
| 19 | 15 | 2 | 2 | 30 |
| 20 | 15 | 1 | 2 | 30 |
| 21 | 30 nonstop | | | 30 |

*Stay at this level as long as necessary.
**Or as long as it takes for you to catch your breath.

From this point on, keep rowing thirty minutes nonstop three
times a week. This schedule assumes you row at least three

**Beginner's Rowing Program,** continued

times a week. If it moves too slowly, promote yourself to the next stage sooner. If it progresses too quickly, remain at each stage for two or three weeks instead of one.

Once you've completed your day's scheduled rowing, you can stay out in the boat practicing for as long as you wish. Just don't overexert.

# Intermediate Rowing

You are an intermediate rower if you can row two and a half or three miles in an hour. This is more than you need to stay in good condition. If you want to learn new techniques or join in regattas or other rowing activities, consider joining a rowing club. Some clubs concentrate on competition, but others assume the role of matchmaker, bringing together student and teacher, rower and boats, rower and rower. They also organize outings to explore interesting and beautiful inlets, bays, lakes, and rivers.

# Masters Rowing

You are a master rower if you can row seven to nine miles nonstop in less than an hour and a half. By now, you're probably in superb condition.

There's no reason to change your rowing schedule just because you've reached the masters level. Rowing at a sweaty pace for a half hour or more without stopping will give you an excellent workout and become an almost meditative experience.

If you are intrigued by the teamwork and competitiveness of racing, contact the United States Rowing Association (see Resources) and ask about their masters category races in your area. Masters races are divided into men's and women's sections, each with its own lightweight and heavyweight divisions. You'll have a choice between sculls and sweeps. In sculls (two-oar rowing), you might race single (just you and the boat) and doubles (two rowers). In sweeps (one-oar rowing), you have a choice among pairs (two rowers), fours, and eights (with or without a coxswain, the strategist, motivator, and leader of each crew).

# The Pitch for Canoeing and Kayaking

If you think rowing across a quiet bay is practically a religious experience, wait until you try canoeing or kayaking. The boats are so streamlined, the paddle strokes so efficient, you barely riffle the water. You are a water bug skimming and skittering across the surface.

We find our thrill paddling gracefully along smooth, quiet lakes, rivers, and bays, feeling the brush of the breeze and the calm of the water. The skills and spills of running rapids and navigating white water appeal to only the few daredevils among us. We prefer safe, simple sorts of canoeing and kayaking.

Canoeing and kayaking are a great deal easier and less demanding than rowing. You paddle on only one side at a time, so you use both arms for one stroke. Even the weakest people can make their boat cut through the water like a knife.

Kayaks almost always look like Eskimo boats. They are closed, pointed vessels with a hatch for your body. Canoes are usually more open. The multiperson canoes look like plastic imitations of the legendary birchbark canoes. Solo canoes look like kayaks with bigger entry hatches. The distinction between kayaks and canoes is currently blurring—there are some fairly open kayaks and some fairly closed canoes. What's more, most canoes nowadays are paddled from a sitting position, like kayaks, rather than from the painful kneeling position that was once the standard. The primary difference between canoes and kayaks today is this: All canoes are paddled with a short, single-bladed oar, and all kayaks are paddled with a long double-bladed oar.

"I've never understood why anyone would want to row when they could kayak instead. You kayak—or canoe—facing forward, so you see where you're going. Rowers face backward so they spend their time looking at where they've been. What's the point of that?"

This last comment comes from Sherri Candini, a nurse who kayaked for the first time ten years ago. She tried it at Sandra's insistence when Sherri complained she couldn't do most exercises and sports because she had suffered from a stress incontinence problem since the birth of her last child. (This problem affects 40% of all women who have given birth.) The first time out in a kayak, Sherri fell in love with the sport. Now, age 58, she spends as much warm-weather time as possible in her red and white kayak exploring the bays and deltas within an easy drive of her house.

"I like touring across long stretches of flat, quiet water much better than I like running rivers," she says. "I've done some white water. It's a challenge and I like the excitement and adventure. I also like to see the look on the faces of those husky young men when they see this white-haired woman go by.

"River running is a real adrenaline rush, but it's like eating a chocolate bar. It's fun while you're doing it, but once you're done, it's as if you never did it. Touring lasts all day, if you want it to, or you can take trips that last a week. On a long trip, you see all kinds of natural wonders, and you meet some wonderful people who live along the water."

Why choose kayaking over canoeing or vice versa? Personal taste, mostly. In a kayak, you feel settled into the water. Some people like sitting low while others prefer the canoe's higher seating position. A canoe paddle requires a bent-arm stroke that some people prefer. Also, you paddle a canoe with several strokes in a row on one side and then several strokes in a row on the other. A kayak paddle requires a straight-arm stroke, one on one side and then, immediately, one stroke on the other side. A canoe, therefore, is more forgiving. A kayak responds to every command, even if you didn't mean it. "A kayak goes where you think," Sherri said. "A canoe goes where you steer."

Canoeing and kayaking do most of the things rowing does for you—they strengthen your heart and lungs, tone your upper-body muscles, and so on, but not quite to the extent rowing does. Figure that when you kayak or canoe for an hour, you get about three-quarters of the aerobic reward you'd get if you were rowing for the same hour. However, neither one does much for your leg muscles because you use your thighs only isometrically, to push against the sides of the boat to stabilize it.

**Don't canoe or kayak without a doctor's approval if** you have epilepsy, Ménière's disease, or chronic back problems.

# Buying and Testing Your Canoeing and Kayaking Equipment

Remember the old-fashioned canvas or wooden canoes you paddled around the lake at Camp Everywhichway? Each spring, one or two were rotted out, and the rest gave you splinters. Today's canoes and kayaks are lighter and more durable—made of aluminum, fiberglass, or plastics so hardy they're actually bulletproof. Canoes come in solo and tandem models—good for touring, fishing, or exploring. Whatever boat you choose, get a seat. Kneeling may give you more power but it's hell on the knees. We also recommend you use a bent-shaft paddle. It's easier on the back and shoulders. Get the right length of paddle: sit down and rest the handle of the paddle on the floor; your nose should be level with the place where the blade attaches to the shaft.

Kayaks are named after the sort of water they're good for. Flat-water, downriver, or touring boats all work admirably for our kind of smooth-water paddling. They move effortlessly in a straight line through large open bodies of water because they're rather flat and have a ridged (or keeled) bottom. Make sure your kayak has adjustable foot pegs so you can move them to accommodate the length of your legs.

Use a light fiberglass paddle; they're infinitely less tiring to maneuver than wood. Ask to try all three grips (right hand, left hand, and universal or ambidextrous). Even if you've never kayaked before, one may feel much more comfortable than another. You may, for example, discover you're a left-handed paddler even though you use your right hand for everything else.

If you don't want your legs wet from the splash of the paddle, use a spray skirt. They are made of plasticized canvas or neoprene; you don them like a skirt, then climb into the boat and hook the entire hem of the skirt over the edge of the hatch of the boat. We prefer the loose, low-tech plasticized canvas over the tight, high-tech neoprene because canvas skirts are much easier to get on and off.

Canoes and kayaks are a little cheaper to buy and a lot easier to rent than rowing shells. (We recommend renting until you're certain you're committed to boating. As we suggested in the rowing section, check your phone book.) Prices range from $250 for sound utilitarian and used models to $1,500 for top-of-the-line boats. Good paddles run anywhere from $80 to $150. Kayaks, especially, are lighter to carry, something to consider if you're going to have to portage (jargon for "carry") them across parking lots or grassy meadows.

## Clothing for Canoeing and Kayaking

In very warm weather, a bathing suit or shorts and a T-shirt—plus a hat, sunglasses, and plenty of sunscreen—are the usual costume for canoeing and kayaking in calm flat water, but wear whatever is comfortable. If the weather is cool, or if you're going out for a long enough period that the weather may change, dress in layers to pile on or peel off and stow in the boat as needed. Include a wool sweater, because wool keeps you fairly warm even when it's wet. Most people don't wear shoes while paddling, although some sort of soft, flexible canvas tie-on footwear comes in handy to protect your feet from rocks or sharp seashells when you're getting in and out of the boat. Don't forget to drink lots of water on hot days, and take a plastic bottle of water with you. Even with a nice breeze off the water, you'll work up enough of a sweat to risk heat injury. See Chapter 4 for more information on protecting yourself from the heat and cold.

Always wear a Coast Guard rated life jacket when you paddle. See the Rowing section for an explanation of the rating system.

## Warming Up for Canoeing and Kayaking

Paddle slowly and gently for five or ten minutes to warm up your heart and loosen your arm and shoulder muscles. When you're done for the day, cool down by paddling around lazily for five or ten minutes before you get out of the boat.

# The Basics of Canoeing and Kayaking

Paddle on calm, flat, predictable water, away from all currents. The slightest turbulence may overturn your boat. Also, paddle parallel to the shore and stay close enough to the beach that someone will see you if you capsize.

## FIVE-MINUTE CANOEING LESSON

We prefer paddling a canoe racing style. That means seated, using a bent-shaft paddle and short, quick strokes. It is easy, fast, and doesn't hurt your shoulders or back.

Put your left hand on the grip and your right hand on the shaft about a foot above the blade. (Reverse the instructions if you're left-handed.) If you've got a bent-shaft paddle, hold it so that its blade is tilted back and down. Swing your right arm forward. In the process, your left hand will come up to shoulder or chin level. Now, slice your paddle into the water and imagine you're holding it there while your body, especially your back, pulls the canoe toward the paddle. Push out and down with your left arm to push the paddle through the water. Drop your left hand to your lap, and your paddle will cut out of the water. Keep paddling on the right side until your canoe starts veering to the left. Then paddle on the other side. Eventually, you'll be able to get six to ten strokes on each side.

## FIVE-MINUTE KAYAKING LESSON

Adjust the footbrace so that your knees are bent and your thighs are snugged in on each side of the hatch. Press out with the knees against the sides of the boat to stabilize it. Grasp the paddle with your hands just a bit wider than shoulder width. Let's say you grip with your right hand. With your right hand, hold the paddle firmly. Let the paddle rotate freely in your left. Now, reach forward and down with your right arm to slice the paddle into the water. Straighten your left arm, directly from the shoulder, as you pull back with your right. The straight-arm push thrusts the paddle through the water more than the other arm pulls. Now, lean forward and dip the paddle on the other side. Alternate sides with every stroke unless you want to turn. Note: Just because you're right-handed doesn't mean you paddle with a right grip. Experiment. One side will feel much more comfortable than the other.

If you ever feel as if you're tipping over, press the blade of your paddle flat against the water the way you'd put out your hand to keep yourself from falling.

## SCHEDULE

Paddle the same way you'd row—paddling and resting, paddling and resting, for as long as you feel like it. Work yourself up to nonstop jaunts of at least a half hour.

Canoes and kayaks are much easier to manipulate than rowing shells. They don't ask you to concentrate on coordinating four different movements at the same time. As a result, you can climb into a canoe or kayak and paddle around the very first day. It will take only a few minutes to get the hang of the paddling techniques; then you can get some exercise and see the sights while you streamline your style.

Start out paddling slow and easy. Whenever you get tired, rest your paddle across the boat and take a breather. Then paddle some more. After your warm-up, paddle hard and fast enough to huff and puff, but not so hard as to get truly winded. As you progress, you'll paddle for longer periods and take shorter rests.

A half hour of huff-and-puff nonstop paddling three times a week is enough for aerobic fitness. If you want to stay out longer, fine, but pace yourself. Either do your thirty minutes workout and then paddle lazily for the rest of the time, or paddle two or three times as long at half or one-third speed. Whatever you do, don't go so far that you have no energy for the return trip. (See Beginner's Canoeing and Kayaking Program on the following page.)

# Intermediate Canoeing and Kayaking

You are an intermediate paddler if you can paddle for an hour nonstop. If your only interest is staying fit and spending some relaxing time out on the water, just continue with your long, steady paddling close and parallel to shore. You'll find it exciting, relaxing, and invigorating to explore inlets, watch the

## BEGINNER'S CANOEING AND
## KAYAKING PROGRAM

| WEEK | PADDLE (IN MINUTES) | REST (IN MINUTES) | REPEATS | TOTAL PADDLING TIME IN MINUTES |
|---|---|---|---|---|
| 1* | at your leisure | at your leisure | | |
| 2 | 5 | 2** | 3 | 15 |
| 3 | 5 | 1 | 3 | 15 |
| 4 | 6 | 2 | 3 | 18 |
| 5 | 6 | 1 | 3 | 18 |
| 6 | 7 | 2 | 3 | 21 |
| 7 | 7 | 1 | 3 | 21 |
| 8 | 8 | 2 | 3 | 24 |
| 9 | 8 | 1 | 3 | 24 |
| 10 | 9 | 2 | 3 | 27 |
| 11 | 9 | 1 | 3 | 27 |
| 12 | 10 | 2 | 3 | 30 |
| 13 | 10 | 1 | 3 | 30 |
| 14 | 15 | 2 | 2 | 30 |
| 15 | 15 | 1 | 2 | 30 |
| 16 | 30 nonstop | | | 30 |

*Stay at this stage until you're comfortable.
**Or as long as it takes for you to catch your breath.

To follow this schedule, paddle at a huff-and-puff pace at least three times a week. If it progresses too quickly, stay at each stage two or three weeks. If it progresses too slowly, either spend only two days (instead of three) at each stage, or eliminate the even-numbered weeks starting with Week 6.

shore birds, or picnic in some quiet cove, while staying in great shape without even thinking about it.

# Masters Canoeing and Kayaking

You are a master paddler if, in addition to paddling one hour nonstop, you know how to read the wind and the water, how to get back into your boat if you capsize in open water, how to use rescue, and other safety techniques. For these and other advanced paddling techniques, you'll need to take lessons. Look under "Boating, Instruction," "Boats, Renting," or "Rafts, Dealers" in the Yellow Pages, or contact the Sierra Club, *Canoe* magazine, or the American Canoe Association for classes near you (see Resources). Until you have these skills, don't even try an otry an open-water trip. It's suicide.

At this point, you may also want to learn how to handle white water (jargon for "rivers with rapids and treacherous currents"). As with open-water paddling, don't even try this unless you've taken classes from qualified instructors in recognizing currents, shallows and depths, and other whims of the water as well as such techniques as the wet exit (getting out of the boat when it's upside down) and an Eskimo roll (turning your boat 360 degrees, from upright through upside down to upright again).

The American Canoeing Association sanctions a variety of canoe and kayak races for all levels of paddlers—novices through Olympic athletes. Among the events are sailing (yes, sailing), flat-water, marathon, wild-water, slalom, canoe poling, and cruising. In general, these races are most popular in states with long traditions of recreational paddling—Maine, California, Wisconsin, and Minnesota—but they're enthusiastically established and available in almost every state.

## SEEING THE WORLD FROM THE WATER

If you're not interested in the thrills and spills (definitely spills) of river running, try touring. If there's an interesting body of quiet water near you, there's sure to be a group that organizes day tours to explore it. It may be anything from a tour of the San Francisco waterfront to island hopping among the tiny islands near Mount Desert in Maine. If that's not enough, you'll find overnight tours up and down some of the major river systems in the United States and Canada. These commercial trips, organized by many of the river rafting tour companies, are about as luxurious as camping out can get. The tour groups provide the guides, the food, the cooks, and usually the canoes or kayaks and all other equipment. And they usually carry all your gear for you, so you have only yourself and your boat to care for. "This ain't roughin' it," Sherri says. "Barbecued chicken or steaks, lots of fresh fruits and vegetables, great cooking. As much as possible, we eat local foods, but we don't have to eat weird things. And none of that freeze-dried junk. This is first-class chow."

# First Aid

Injuries from rowing with a sliding seat or from flat-water canoeing and kayaking are very, very rare.

**Backache:** Occasionally, rowing may cause backache or aggravate an already bad back, but you can prevent this by not leaning back as far when you pull, or leaning back farther, or not rounding your back as much before hitting the catch. To prevent canoeing backaches, kneel on a cushioned pad instead of sitting. Or sit instead of kneeling. Try to keep your back straight; don't round your shoulders; use your whole trunk from the waist up to stroke; reach out with the shoulder, not just with the arm. To prevent kayaking backaches, lean back more as you paddle; bring your footbrace closer so your knees are more bent; or move your footbrace farther back so your knees are a bit straighter. Do sit-downs (See No-Stretch Super Stretches, Chapter 3) to strengthen your abdominal muscles.

**Pain in hands, especially from arthritis:** Pad and thicken the oar grips with strips of foam.

**Blisters:** These are a fact of life during the first few weeks of rowing and also occur, although less often, when paddling. Take heart. After a few weeks, your hands will toughen up. Meanwhile, see the First Aid section in Chapter 8 for home treatment.

You'll never forget your first day on the water. Your movements are strangely soft and quite compelling. Soon, boating becomes a meditative exercise in moving and being moved. And because it's a nonjarring, seated activity, you have found an escape from life that will last a lifetime. Twenty or thirty years from now, look around. We may be coming up on your tail. Until then, keep on moving and have a ball.

# R E S O U R C E S

**GENERAL**
**Books**

*Arthritis. A Comprehensive Guide,* Dr. James F. Fries, Addison-Wesley, 1979. All health books should be written this clearly and as loaded with information. Covers every aspect of arthritis and includes numerous charts for diagnosing what sort of arthritis you have and how to treat it.

*The Diabetic's Sports and Exercise Book,* June Bierman and Barbara Toohey, J. B. Lippincott Company, 1977. Still the only thorough, reliable book for the diabetic on how to exercise; how to adjust your insulin; how to eat before, during, and after exercise; how to dress; how to take care of your feet; how to . . . just about everything.

*Rhymes to Predict the Weather,* Don Haggerty, SpringMeadow Publishers, P.O. Box 31038, Seattle, Wash. 98103. Since we've been exercising, we've become interested in the weather—the different kinds of clouds, which wind brings what kind of weather, how to know when a front is passing through and the weather is about to change. This charming, unassuming little book teaches weather prediction to nonscientists through pithy, sometimes corny jingles.

**WALKING**
**Magazines and Books**

*The Walking Magazine,* 711 Boylston St., Boston, Mass. 02116.

*Walk Ways/Walking Journal,* Walk, Inc., 733 Fifteenth St. N.W., Suite 427, Washington, D.C. 20005.

*The Complete Book of Exercisewalking,* Gary Yanker, Contemporary Books, Chicago, 1983. Much better organized and more thorough than the new edition.

*Race Walking: A Safe and Healthy Alternative to Jogging,* William Finley and Marion Weinstein, Stephen Greene Press, Lexington, Mass., 1985.

*On Foot Through Europe Trail Guides,* available from Whole Earth Access Company, 2990 Seventh St., Berkeley, Calif. 94710. Regions include Europe's Long Trails; the British Isles; West Germany; Scandinavia; France and Benelux nations; Spain and Portugal; Austria and Switzerland.

*Be Expert with Map and Compass,* Bjorn Kjellstrom, available from Klutz, P.O. Box 2992, Stanford, Calif. 94305. The classic on orienteering, by *the* authority. Explains how to make sense of a topographical map, how to get where you want to go and home again. Silva orienteering compass included.

**Organizations**

The Walkers Center, 733 Fifteenth St. N.W., Suite 427, Washington, D.C. 20005.

Sierra Club, 530 Bush St., San Francisco, Calif. 94108.

Walkers Club of America, 445 East 86th St., New York, N.Y. 10028. Race walking competition clearinghouse.

U.S. Orienteering Federation, P.O. Box 1039, Ballwin, Mo. 63011.

Also check with your local heritage, cultural, architectural, and historical societies; the YMCA; local chapter of the American Heart Association (they often sponsor Heart and Sole Walks); and check out anything called a volksmarch, a name reserved for organized but noncompetitive walks.


# RUNNING
## Books

*Galloway's Book on Running,* Jeff Galloway, Shelter Publications, Inc., Bolinas, Calif., 1984.


# SWIMMING
## Magazines and Books

*Swim-Master,* 2308 Northeast Nineteenth Ave., Fort Lauderdale, Fla. 33305.

*Swim Swim,* P.O. Box 5901, Santa Monica, Calif. 90405.

*The Fit Swimmer: 120 Workouts and Training Tips,* Marianne Brems, Contemporary Books, Chicago, 1984.

*I Can Swim, You Can Swim,* Tom Cuthbertson and Lee Cole, Ten Speed Press, Berkeley, Calif., 1979.

*Total Swimming,* Harvey S. Weiner, Simon and Schuster, New York, 1980.

*Water Workout: 120 Water Exercises for Swimmers and Nonswimmers,* Bill Reed and Murray Rose, Harmony Books, New York, 1985.

*The W.E.T. Workout,* Jane Katz, Facts on File, 1985.

**Organizations**

U.S. Masters Swimming, c/o Dorothy Donnelly, 5 Piggott Lane, Avon, Conn. 06001. The national competitive network for swimmers over the age of nineteen.

Masters Swimming Program, F. H. Haartz, Chairman, 155 Pantry Rd., Sudbury, Mass. 10776. Events for people over forty.

Senior Olympics/Senior Sports International Association, 5670 Wilshire Blvd., Suite 360, Los Angeles, Calif. 90036.

National Institute for Creative Aquatics, Elaine Douma, President, 12 Washington Lane, West Milford, N.J. 07480.

Amateur Athletic Union, Water Polo, U.S. National Sports Building, 1750 East Boulder St., Colorado Springs, Colo. 80909.

International Swimming Hall of Fame, 1 Hall of Fame Drive, Fort Lauderdale, Fla. 33316. Great resource center; library, bookstore.

**Mail Order**

*Powerstroke gloves:* Early Winters, 110 Prefontaine Place South, Seattle, Wash. 08104.

*The Wet Vest* (an exercise vest for water aerobics): Bioenergetics, Inc., 5074 Shelby Drive, Birmingham, Ala. 35243.

Check the ads in *Swim Swim* for other equipment.


**CYCLING**

**Magazines and Books**

*Bicycling,* Emmaus, Pa. 18049. Magazine devoted to all aspects of cycling. Offers tips for beginners, best-buy ratings of bikes and related equipment, as well as technical how-to's on repairs and customizing bikes.

*Anybody's Bike Book: An Original Manual of Bike Repairs,* Tom Cuthbertson, Ten Speed Press, Berkeley, Calif. The simplest, all-the-beginner-needs-to-know instruction book on the market.

*Bicycling,* John Marino, Jeremy P. Tarcher, Inc., Los Angeles, 1981.

*Bike Touring: The Sierra Club Guide to Outings on Wheels,* Raymond Bridge, Sierra Club Books, San Francisco, 1979.

**Organizations**

Bikecentennial, P.O. Box 8308, Missoula, Mont. 59807. *The* nonprofit, member-supported service organization for touring bicyclists.

**Mail Order**

*Instant Tandem attachment:* Instant Tandem Co. Inc., 1307 Kirkland Ave., Kirkland, Wash. 98033.

*Whistle pedaling canoe:* SaberCraft, 1501 West Dry Creek Rd., Healdsburg, Calif. 95448.

## CROSS-COUNTRY SKIING
### Magazines and Books
*Cross Country Skier,* P.O. Box 1203, West Brattleboro, Vt. 05301.
### Organizations
U.S. Ski Association, U.S. Olympic Complex, 1750 East Boulder St., Colorado Springs, Colo. 80909. Governing body for competitive amateur Nordic and Alpine skiing.

Ski Touring Council, West Hill Rd., Troy, Vt. 05868. Promotes noncompetitive cross-country skiing.

## ROWING, CANOEING, AND KAYAKING
### Magazines
*Canoe,* P.O. Box 10748, Des Moines, Iowa 50340. Devoted to all forms of canoeing and kayaking; includes consumer buying information, travel features, and articles on technique.

*Sea Kayaker,* 6327 Seaview Ave. N.W., Seattle, Wash. 98107.
### Organizations
U.S. Rowing Association, 251 North Illinois, #980, Indianapolis, Ind. 46204.

The Sierra Club, 530 Bush St., San Francisco, Calif. 94108.

American Canoe Association, P.O. Box 248, Lorton, Va. 22079. Organization for canoeists and kayakers at every level of skill. Sanctions races, provides educational and training services, works toward conservation of waterways. Member of U.S. Olympic Committee.

U.S. Canoe Association, 617 South 94th St., Milwaukee, Wis. 53214.
### Suppliers
*Rowing catamaran:* Rowcat, Art Javes Designs, Ltd., 4914 Seventeenth Ave. S., Gulfport, Fla. 33707.

*Rowing catamaran:* Omni-Cat Designs, 715 Emory Valley Rd., Oak Ridge, Tenn. 37830.

*Classic recreational rowing shell:* Alden Shells, Martin Marine Co., P.O. Box 2510, Goodwin Rd., Kittery Point, Maine 03905.

*Classic recreational rowing shell and short double scull:* Laser West, 1769 Placentia Ave., Costa Mesa, Calif. 92627.

*Handmade kayaks, canoes, and sailing kayaks:* Baldwin Boat Company, Hoxie Hill Rd., Orrington, Maine 04474. These don't look like the high-tech, sexy things you see at boat shows, but they are *the* kayaks that go where you think. Every boat made completely by hand by Earl Baldwin. Sandra's favorite downriver or touring kayak. We mention this mail-order source because you'll never find these boats in a store.

# I N D E X

Abdominal muscles, 31–32
Achilles tendinitis, 63
Adenosine triphosphate (ATP), 14
Aerobic exercise. *See also*
    Indoor exercise; Outdoor
    exercise; *and names of*
    *activities*
  benefits of, 3, 4–5, 6–9, 11,
    13–21
  classes, 11
  defined, 12
  high-impact, 11–12
  low-impact, 12
  recommended amounts of,
    23–24
  time spent, 20–21
Aging, 5–6, 41
Air temperature, and humidity,
  42–43
Alcoholic beverages, 44, 47

Allergies, 67–68
Amateur Athletic Union, Water
  Polo section, 171
American Canoeing Association,
  224
American College of Sports
  Medicine, 22–23
Angina, 38
Ankles, and rope skipping, 129
Anxiety. *See* Stress reduction
Appetite, 17
Aquaerobics, 170
Arteries, 5, 7
Arthritis, 9, 62–67
  cross-country skiing machines
    and, 109
  defined, 63
  exercising with, 66–67
  home treatment, 64, 65–67
  most common kinds, 63–64
  when to see doctor, 64–65

# ABOUT THE AUTHORS

RONALD M. LAWRENCE, M.D., Ph.D., is known throughout the world as one of the original sports medicine pioneers as well as an innovator in treating chronic pain.

He is president of the American Running and Fitness Association, chairman of sports medicine of the Amateur Athletic Union of the United States, and medical director of the AAU Master's Program, the organization that supports and runs local and national races, meets, and competitions for amateur athletes over the age of forty. He is a former consultant to the U.S. Olympic Committee's Sports Medicine Council, president and founder of the American Medical Athletics Association, secretary of the American Academy of Sports Physicians, and former member of the National Advisory Council on Aging of the National Institutes of Health.

In addition to his private practice in neurology, focusing on healing people with chronic pain problems, he is assistant clinical professor at the Neuropsychiatric Institute, UCLA School of Medicine, and director of the Western Geriatric Research Institute. Using exercise and other techniques, he has liberated countless patients from the agony of arthritis and back and neck pain and has taught other patients with intractable pain how to alleviate it and move around again.

SANDRA ROSENZWEIG, a zoologist and anthropologist, has been a medical writer for almost twenty years. Her articles are published in most major national magazines; her *Sportsfitness* column is syndicated to newspapers all over the United States; and her *Sportsfitness for Women* has become a standard of the field—a complete resource book for women of all ages (childhood through very old age) and all levels of devotion to exercise.

She designs exercise programs for industry and private groups and organizes seminars and workshops on fitness and current health issues for nonprofit groups. She also works as a consultant with physicians in San Francisco, Los Angeles, and New York to create exercise programs for patients with specific medical problems or sports injuries.